FREE Study Skills Videos ~~√D~~ Offer

Dear Customer,

Thank you for your purchase from Mometrix! We consider it an honor and a privilege that you have purchased our product and we want to ensure your satisfaction.

As a way of showing our appreciation and to help us better serve you, we have developed Study Skills Videos that we would like to give you for <u>FREE</u>. These videos cover our *best practices* for getting ready for your exam, from how to use our study materials to how to best prepare for the day of the test.

All that we ask is that you email us with feedback that would describe your experience so far with our product. Good, bad, or indifferent, we want to know what you think!

To get your FREE Study Skills Videos, you can use the **QR code** below, or send us an **email** at <u>studyvideos@mometrix.com</u> with *FREE VIDEOS* in the subject line and the following information in the body of the email:

- The name of the product you purchased.
- Your product rating on a scale of 1-5, with 5 being the highest rating.
- Your feedback. It can be long, short, or anything in between. We just want to know your impressions and experience so far with our product. (Good feedback might include how our study material met your needs and ways we might be able to make it even better. You could highlight features that you found helpful or features that you think we should add.)

If you have any questions or concerns, please don't hesitate to contact me directly.

Thanks again!

Sincerely,

Jay Willis
Vice President
<u>jay.willis@mometrix.com</u>
1-800-673-8175

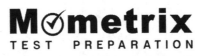

Medical Technologist Exam
SECRETS

Study Guide
Your Key to Exam Success

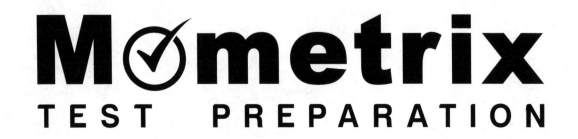

Written and edited by the Mometrix Medical Laboratory Certification Test Team

Printed in the United States of America

This paper meets the requirements of ANSI/NISO Z39.48-1992 (Permanence of Paper).

Mometrix offers volume discount pricing to institutions. For more information or a price quote, please contact our sales department at sales@mometrix.com or 888-248-1219.

Paperback
ISBN 13: 978-1-61072-011-3
ISBN 10: 1-61072-011-3

Ebook
ISBN 13: 978-1-62120-589-0
ISBN 10: 1-62120-589-4

DEAR FUTURE EXAM SUCCESS STORY

First of all, **THANK YOU** for purchasing Mometrix study materials!

Second, congratulations! You are one of the few determined test-takers who are committed to doing whatever it takes to excel on your exam. **You have come to the right place.** We developed these study materials with one goal in mind: to deliver you the information you need in a format that's concise and easy to use.

In addition to optimizing your guide for the content of the test, we've outlined our recommended steps for breaking down the preparation process into small, attainable goals so you can make sure you stay on track.

We've also analyzed the entire test-taking process, identifying the most common pitfalls and showing how you can overcome them and be ready for any curveball the test throws you.

Standardized testing is one of the biggest obstacles on your road to success, which only increases the importance of doing well in the high-pressure, high-stakes environment of test day. Your results on this test could have a significant impact on your future, and this guide provides the information and practical advice to help you achieve your full potential on test day.

Your success is our success

We would love to hear from you! If you would like to share the story of your exam success or if you have any questions or comments in regard to our products, please contact us at **800-673-8175** or **support@mometrix.com**.

Thanks again for your business and we wish you continued success!

Sincerely,
The Mometrix Test Preparation Team

> **Need more help? Check out our flashcards at:**
> **http://mometrixflashcards.com/MedicalTechnologist**

TABLE OF CONTENTS

Introduction

Thank you for purchasing this resource! You have made the choice to prepare yourself for a test that could have a huge impact on your future, and this guide is designed to help you be fully ready for test day. Obviously, it's important to have a solid understanding of the test material, but you also need to be prepared for the unique environment and stressors of the test, so that you can perform to the best of your abilities.

For this purpose, the first section that appears in this guide is the **Secret Keys**. We've devoted countless hours to meticulously researching what works and what doesn't, and we've boiled down our findings to the five most impactful steps you can take to improve your performance on the test. We start at the beginning with study planning and move through the preparation process, all the way to the testing strategies that will help you get the most out of what you know when you're finally sitting in front of the test.

We recommend that you start preparing for your test as far in advance as possible. However, if you've bought this guide as a last-minute study resource and only have a few days before your test, we recommend that you skip over the first two Secret Keys since they address a long-term study plan.

If you struggle with **test anxiety**, we strongly encourage you to check out our recommendations for how you can overcome it. Test anxiety is a formidable foe, but it can be beaten, and we want to make sure you have the tools you need to defeat it.

Secret Key #1 – Plan Big, Study Small

There's a lot riding on your performance. If you want to ace this test, you're going to need to keep your skills sharp and the material fresh in your mind. You need a plan that lets you review everything you need to know while still fitting in your schedule. We'll break this strategy down into three categories.

Information Organization

Start with the information you already have: the official test outline. From this, you can make a complete list of all the concepts you need to cover before the test. Organize these concepts into groups that can be studied together, and create a list of any related vocabulary you need to learn so you can brush up on any difficult terms. You'll want to keep this vocabulary list handy once you actually start studying since you may need to add to it along the way.

Time Management

Once you have your set of study concepts, decide how to spread them out over the time you have left before the test. Break your study plan into small, clear goals so you have a manageable task for each day and know exactly what you're doing. Then just focus on one small step at a time. When you manage your time this way, you don't need to spend hours at a time studying. Studying a small block of content for a short period each day helps you retain information better and avoid stressing over how much you have left to do. You can relax knowing that you have a plan to cover everything in time. In order for this strategy to be effective though, you have to start studying early and stick to your schedule. Avoid the exhaustion and futility that comes from last-minute cramming!

Study Environment

The environment you study in has a big impact on your learning. Studying in a coffee shop, while probably more enjoyable, is not likely to be as fruitful as studying in a quiet room. It's important to keep distractions to a minimum. You're only planning to study for a short block of time, so make the most of it. Don't pause to check your phone or get up to find a snack. It's also important to **avoid multitasking**. Research has consistently shown that multitasking will make your studying dramatically less effective. Your study area should also be comfortable and well-lit so you don't have the distraction of straining your eyes or sitting on an uncomfortable chair.

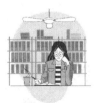 The time of day you study is also important. You want to be rested and alert. Don't wait until just before bedtime. Study when you'll be most likely to comprehend and remember. Even better, if you know what time of day your test will be, set that time aside for study. That way your brain will be used to working on that subject at that specific time and you'll have a better chance of recalling information.

Finally, it can be helpful to team up with others who are studying for the same test. Your actual studying should be done in as isolated an environment as possible, but the work of organizing the information and setting up the study plan can be divided up. In between study sessions, you can discuss with your teammates the concepts that you're all studying and quiz each other on the details. Just be sure that your teammates are as serious about the test as you are. If you find that your study time is being replaced with social time, you might need to find a new team.

2

Secret Key #2 – Make Your Studying Count

You're devoting a lot of time and effort to preparing for this test, so you want to be absolutely certain it will pay off. This means doing more than just reading the content and hoping you can remember it on test day. It's important to make every minute of study count. There are two main areas you can focus on to make your studying count.

Retention

It doesn't matter how much time you study if you can't remember the material. You need to make sure you are retaining the concepts. To check your retention of the information you're learning, try recalling it at later times with minimal prompting. Try carrying around flashcards and glance at one or two from time to time or ask a friend who's also studying for the test to quiz you.

To enhance your retention, look for ways to put the information into practice so that you can apply it rather than simply recalling it. If you're using the information in practical ways, it will be much easier to remember. Similarly, it helps to solidify a concept in your mind if you're not only reading it to yourself but also explaining it to someone else. Ask a friend to let you teach them about a concept you're a little shaky on (or speak aloud to an imaginary audience if necessary). As you try to summarize, define, give examples, and answer your friend's questions, you'll understand the concepts better and they will stay with you longer. Finally, step back for a big picture view and ask yourself how each piece of information fits with the whole subject. When you link the different concepts together and see them working together as a whole, it's easier to remember the individual components.

Finally, practice showing your work on any multi-step problems, even if you're just studying. Writing out each step you take to solve a problem will help solidify the process in your mind, and you'll be more likely to remember it during the test.

Modality

Modality simply refers to the means or method by which you study. Choosing a study modality that fits your own individual learning style is crucial. No two people learn best in exactly the same way, so it's important to know your strengths and use them to your advantage.

For example, if you learn best by visualization, focus on visualizing a concept in your mind and draw an image or a diagram. Try color-coding your notes, illustrating them, or creating symbols that will trigger your mind to recall a learned concept. If you learn best by hearing or discussing information, find a study partner who learns the same way or read aloud to yourself. Think about how to put the information in your own words. Imagine that you are giving a lecture on the topic and record yourself so you can listen to it later.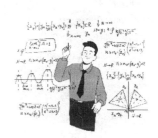

For any learning style, flashcards can be helpful. Organize the information so you can take advantage of spare moments to review. Underline key words or phrases. Use different colors for different categories. Mnemonic devices (such as creating a short list in which every item starts with the same letter) can also help with retention. Find what works best for you and use it to store the information in your mind most effectively and easily.

3

Secret Key #3 – Practice the Right Way

Your success on test day depends not only on how many hours you put into preparing, but also on whether you prepared the right way. It's good to check along the way to see if your studying is paying off. One of the most effective ways to do this is by taking practice tests to evaluate your progress. Practice tests are useful because they show exactly where you need to improve. Every time you take a practice test, pay special attention to these three groups of questions:

- The questions you got wrong
- The questions you had to guess on, even if you guessed right
- The questions you found difficult or slow to work through

This will show you exactly what your weak areas are, and where you need to devote more study time. Ask yourself why each of these questions gave you trouble. Was it because you didn't understand the material? Was it because you didn't remember the vocabulary? Do you need more repetitions on this type of question to build speed and confidence? Dig into those questions and figure out how you can strengthen your weak areas as you go back to review the material.

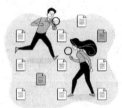 Additionally, many practice tests have a section explaining the answer choices. It can be tempting to read the explanation and think that you now have a good understanding of the concept. However, an explanation likely only covers part of the question's broader context. Even if the explanation makes perfect sense, **go back and investigate** every concept related to the question until you're positive you have a thorough understanding.

As you go along, keep in mind that the practice test is just that: practice. Memorizing these questions and answers will not be very helpful on the actual test because it is unlikely to have any of the same exact questions. If you only know the right answers to the sample questions, you won't be prepared for the real thing. **Study the concepts** until you understand them fully, and then you'll be able to answer any question that shows up on the test.

It's important to wait on the practice tests until you're ready. If you take a test on your first day of study, you may be overwhelmed by the amount of material covered and how much you need to learn. Work up to it gradually.

On test day, you'll need to be prepared for answering questions, managing your time, and using the test-taking strategies you've learned. It's a lot to balance, like a mental marathon that will have a big impact on your future. Like training for a marathon, you'll need to start slowly and work your way up. When test day arrives, you'll be ready.

Start with the strategies you've read in the first two Secret Keys—plan your course and study in the way that works best for you. If you have time, consider using multiple study resources to get different approaches to the same concepts. It can be helpful to see difficult concepts from more than one angle. Then find a good source for practice tests. Many times, the test website will suggest potential study resources or provide sample tests.

Practice Test Strategy

If you're able to find at least three practice tests, we recommend this strategy:

UNTIMED AND OPEN-BOOK PRACTICE

Take the first test with no time constraints and with your notes and study guide handy. Take your time and focus on applying the strategies you've learned.

TIMED AND OPEN-BOOK PRACTICE

Take the second practice test open-book as well, but set a timer and practice pacing yourself to finish in time.

TIMED AND CLOSED-BOOK PRACTICE

Take any other practice tests as if it were test day. Set a timer and put away your study materials. Sit at a table or desk in a quiet room, imagine yourself at the testing center, and answer questions as quickly and accurately as possible.

Keep repeating timed and closed-book tests on a regular basis until you run out of practice tests or it's time for the actual test. Your mind will be ready for the schedule and stress of test day, and you'll be able to focus on recalling the material you've learned.

Secret Key #4 – Pace Yourself

Once you're fully prepared for the material on the test, your biggest challenge on test day will be managing your time. Just knowing that the clock is ticking can make you panic even if you have plenty of time left. Work on pacing yourself so you can build confidence against the time constraints of the exam. Pacing is a difficult skill to master, especially in a high-pressure environment, so **practice is vital**.

Set time expectations for your pace based on how much time is available. For example, if a section has 60 questions and the time limit is 30 minutes, you know you have to average 30 seconds or less per question in order to answer them all. Although 30 seconds is the hard limit, set 25 seconds per question as your goal, so you reserve extra time to spend on harder questions. When you budget extra time for the harder questions, you no longer have any reason to stress when those questions take longer to answer.

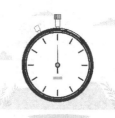

Don't let this time expectation distract you from working through the test at a calm, steady pace, but keep it in mind so you don't spend too much time on any one question. Recognize that taking extra time on one question you don't understand may keep you from answering two that you do understand later in the test. If your time limit for a question is up and you're still not sure of the answer, mark it and move on, and come back to it later if the time and the test format allow. If the testing format doesn't allow you to return to earlier questions, just make an educated guess; then put it out of your mind and move on.

On the easier questions, be careful not to rush. It may seem wise to hurry through them so you have more time for the challenging ones, but it's not worth missing one if you know the concept and just didn't take the time to read the question fully. Work efficiently but make sure you understand the question and have looked at all of the answer choices, since more than one may seem right at first.

Even if you're paying attention to the time, you may find yourself a little behind at some point. You should speed up to get back on track, but do so wisely. Don't panic; just take a few seconds less on each question until you're caught up. Don't guess without thinking, but do look through the answer choices and eliminate any you know are wrong. If you can get down to two choices, it is often worthwhile to guess from those. Once you've chosen an answer, move on and don't dwell on any that you skipped or had to hurry through. If a question was taking too long, chances are it was one of the harder ones, so you weren't as likely to get it right anyway.

On the other hand, if you find yourself getting ahead of schedule, it may be beneficial to slow down a little. The more quickly you work, the more likely you are to make a careless mistake that will affect your score. You've budgeted time for each question, so don't be afraid to spend that time. Practice an efficient but careful pace to get the most out of the time you have.

Secret Key #5 – Have a Plan for Guessing

When you're taking the test, you may find yourself stuck on a question. Some of the answer choices seem better than others, but you don't see the one answer choice that is obviously correct. What do you do?

The scenario described above is very common, yet most test takers have not effectively prepared for it. Developing and practicing a plan for guessing may be one of the single most effective uses of your time as you get ready for the exam.

In developing your plan for guessing, there are three questions to address:

- When should you start the guessing process?
- How should you narrow down the choices?
- Which answer should you choose?

When to Start the Guessing Process

Unless your plan for guessing is to select C every time (which, despite its merits, is not what we recommend), you need to leave yourself enough time to apply your answer elimination strategies. Since you have a limited amount of time for each question, that means that if you're going to give yourself the best shot at guessing correctly, you have to decide quickly whether or not you will guess.

Of course, the best-case scenario is that you don't have to guess at all, so first, see if you can answer the question based on your knowledge of the subject and basic reasoning skills. Focus on the key words in the question and try to jog your memory of related topics. Give yourself a chance to bring the knowledge to mind, but once you realize that you don't have (or you can't access) the knowledge you need to answer the question, it's time to start the guessing process.

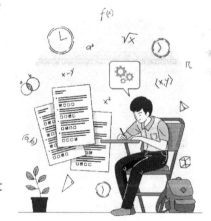

It's almost always better to start the guessing process too early than too late. It only takes a few seconds to remember something and answer the question from knowledge. Carefully eliminating wrong answer choices takes longer. Plus, going through the process of eliminating answer choices can actually help jog your memory.

Summary: Start the guessing process as soon as you decide that you can't answer the question based on your knowledge.

7

How to Narrow Down the Choices

The next chapter in this book (**Test-Taking Strategies**) includes a wide range of strategies for how to approach questions and how to look for answer choices to eliminate. You will definitely want to read those carefully, practice them, and figure out which ones work best for you. Here though, we're going to address a mindset rather than a particular strategy.

Your odds of guessing an answer correctly depend on how many options you are choosing from.

Number of options left	5	4	3	2	1
Odds of guessing correctly	20%	25%	33%	50%	100%

You can see from this chart just how valuable it is to be able to eliminate incorrect answers and make an educated guess, but there are two things that many test takers do that cause them to miss out on the benefits of guessing:

- Accidentally eliminating the correct answer
- Selecting an answer based on an impression

We'll look at the first one here, and the second one in the next section.

To avoid accidentally eliminating the correct answer, we recommend a thought exercise called **the $5 challenge**. In this challenge, you only eliminate an answer choice from contention if you are willing to bet $5 on it being wrong. Why $5? Five dollars is a small but not insignificant amount of money. It's an amount you could afford to lose but wouldn't want to throw away. And while losing

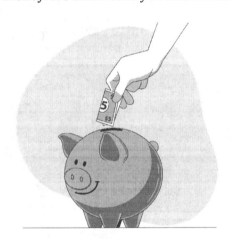

$5 once might not hurt too much, doing it twenty times will set you back $100. In the same way, each small decision you make—eliminating a choice here, guessing on a question there—won't by itself impact your score very much, but when you put them all together, they can make a big difference. By holding each answer choice elimination decision to a higher standard, you can reduce the risk of accidentally eliminating the correct answer.

The $5 challenge can also be applied in a positive sense: If you are willing to bet $5 that an answer choice *is* correct, go ahead and mark it as correct.

Summary: Only eliminate an answer choice if you are willing to bet $5 that it is wrong.

Which Answer to Choose

You're taking the test. You've run into a hard question and decided you'll have to guess. You've eliminated all the answer choices you're willing to bet $5 on. Now you have to pick an answer. Why do we even need to talk about this? Why can't you just pick whichever one you feel like when the time comes?

The answer to these questions is that if you don't come into the test with a plan, you'll rely on your impression to select an answer choice, and if you do that, you risk falling into a trap. The test writers know that everyone who takes their test will be guessing on some of the questions, so they intentionally write wrong answer choices to seem plausible. You still have to pick an answer though, and if the wrong answer choices are designed to look right, how can you ever be sure that you're not falling for their trap? The best solution we've found to this dilemma is to take the decision out of your hands entirely. Here is the process we recommend:

Once you've eliminated any choices that you are confident (willing to bet $5) are wrong, select the first remaining choice as your answer.

Whether you choose to select the first remaining choice, the second, or the last, the important thing is that you use some preselected standard. Using this approach guarantees that you will not be enticed into selecting an answer choice that looks right, because you are not basing your decision on how the answer choices look.

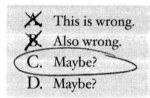

This is not meant to make you question your knowledge. Instead, it is to help you recognize the difference between your knowledge and your impressions. There's a huge difference between thinking an answer is right because of what you know, and thinking an answer is right because it looks or sounds like it should be right.

Summary: To ensure that your selection is appropriately random, make a predetermined selection from among all answer choices you have not eliminated.

Test-Taking Strategies

This section contains a list of test-taking strategies that you may find helpful as you work through the test. By taking what you know and applying logical thought, you can maximize your chances of answering any question correctly!

It is very important to realize that every question is different and every person is different: no single strategy will work on every question, and no single strategy will work for every person. That's why we've included all of them here, so you can try them out and determine which ones work best for different types of questions and which ones work best for you.

Question Strategies

☑ READ CAREFULLY

Read the question and the answer choices carefully. Don't miss the question because you misread the terms. You have plenty of time to read each question thoroughly and make sure you understand what is being asked. Yet a happy medium must be attained, so don't waste too much time. You must read carefully and efficiently.

☑ CONTEXTUAL CLUES

Look for contextual clues. If the question includes a word you are not familiar with, look at the immediate context for some indication of what the word might mean. Contextual clues can often give you all the information you need to decipher the meaning of an unfamiliar word. Even if you can't determine the meaning, you may be able to narrow down the possibilities enough to make a solid guess at the answer to the question.

☑ PREFIXES

If you're having trouble with a word in the question or answer choices, try dissecting it. Take advantage of every clue that the word might include. Prefixes and suffixes can be a huge help. Usually, they allow you to determine a basic meaning. *Pre-* means before, *post-* means after, *pro-* is positive, *de-* is negative. From prefixes and suffixes, you can get an idea of the general meaning of the word and try to put it into context.

☑ HEDGE WORDS

Watch out for critical hedge words, such as *likely, may, can, sometimes, often, almost, mostly, usually, generally, rarely*, and *sometimes*. Question writers insert these hedge phrases to cover every possibility. Often an answer choice will be wrong simply because it leaves no room for exception. Be on guard for answer choices that have definitive words such as *exactly* and *always*.

☑ SWITCHBACK WORDS

Stay alert for *switchbacks*. These are the words and phrases frequently used to alert you to shifts in thought. The most common switchback words are *but, although*, and *however*. Others include *nevertheless, on the other hand, even though, while, in spite of, despite*, and *regardless of*. Switchback words are important to catch because they can change the direction of the question or an answer choice.

⊘ Face Value

When in doubt, use common sense. Accept the situation in the problem at face value. Don't read too much into it. These problems will not require you to make wild assumptions. If you have to go beyond creativity and warp time or space in order to have an answer choice fit the question, then you should move on and consider the other answer choices. These are normal problems rooted in reality. The applicable relationship or explanation may not be readily apparent, but it is there for you to figure out. Use your common sense to interpret anything that isn't clear.

Answer Choice Strategies

⊘ Answer Selection

The most thorough way to pick an answer choice is to identify and eliminate wrong answers until only one is left, then confirm it is the correct answer. Sometimes an answer choice may immediately seem right, but be careful. The test writers will usually put more than one reasonable answer choice on each question, so take a second to read all of them and make sure that the other choices are not equally obvious. As long as you have time left, it is better to read every answer choice than to pick the first one that looks right without checking the others.

⊘ Answer Choice Families

An answer choice family consists of two (in rare cases, three) answer choices that are very similar in construction and cannot all be true at the same time. If you see two answer choices that are direct opposites or parallels, one of them is usually the correct answer. For instance, if one answer choice says that quantity x increases and another either says that quantity x decreases (opposite) or says that quantity y increases (parallel), then those answer choices would fall into the same family. An answer choice that doesn't match the construction of the answer choice family is more likely to be incorrect. Most questions will not have answer choice families, but when they do appear, you should be prepared to recognize them.

⊘ Eliminate Answers

Eliminate answer choices as soon as you realize they are wrong, but make sure you consider all possibilities. If you are eliminating answer choices and realize that the last one you are left with is also wrong, don't panic. Start over and consider each choice again. There may be something you missed the first time that you will realize on the second pass.

⊘ Avoid Fact Traps

Don't be distracted by an answer choice that is factually true but doesn't answer the question. You are looking for the choice that answers the question. Stay focused on what the question is asking for so you don't accidentally pick an answer that is true but incorrect. Always go back to the question and make sure the answer choice you've selected actually answers the question and is not merely a true statement.

⊘ Extreme Statements

In general, you should avoid answers that put forth extreme actions as standard practice or proclaim controversial ideas as established fact. An answer choice that states the "process should be used in certain situations, if..." is much more likely to be correct than one that states the "process should be discontinued completely." The first is a calm rational statement and doesn't even make a definitive, uncompromising stance, using a hedge word *if* to provide wiggle room, whereas the second choice is far more extreme.

11

⏀ BENCHMARK

As you read through the answer choices and you come across one that seems to answer the question well, mentally select that answer choice. This is not your final answer, but it's the one that will help you evaluate the other answer choices. The one that you selected is your benchmark or standard for judging each of the other answer choices. Every other answer choice must be compared to your benchmark. That choice is correct until proven otherwise by another answer choice beating it. If you find a better answer, then that one becomes your new benchmark. Once you've decided that no other choice answers the question as well as your benchmark, you have your final answer.

⏀ PREDICT THE ANSWER

Before you even start looking at the answer choices, it is often best to try to predict the answer. When you come up with the answer on your own, it is easier to avoid distractions and traps because you will know exactly what to look for. The right answer choice is unlikely to be word-for-word what you came up with, but it should be a close match. Even if you are confident that you have the right answer, you should still take the time to read each option before moving on.

General Strategies

⏀ TOUGH QUESTIONS

If you are stumped on a problem or it appears too hard or too difficult, don't waste time. Move on! Remember though, if you can quickly check for obviously incorrect answer choices, your chances of guessing correctly are greatly improved. Before you completely give up, at least try to knock out a couple of possible answers. Eliminate what you can and then guess at the remaining answer choices before moving on.

⏀ CHECK YOUR WORK

Since you will probably not know every term listed and the answer to every question, it is important that you get credit for the ones that you do know. Don't miss any questions through careless mistakes. If at all possible, try to take a second to look back over your answer selection and make sure you've selected the correct answer choice and haven't made a costly careless mistake (such as marking an answer choice that you didn't mean to mark). This quick double check should more than pay for itself in caught mistakes for the time it costs.

⏀ PACE YOURSELF

It's easy to be overwhelmed when you're looking at a page full of questions; your mind is confused and full of random thoughts, and the clock is ticking down faster than you would like. Calm down and maintain the pace that you have set for yourself. Especially as you get down to the last few minutes of the test, don't let the small numbers on the clock make you panic. As long as you are on track by monitoring your pace, you are guaranteed to have time for each question.

⏀ DON'T RUSH

It is very easy to make errors when you are in a hurry. Maintaining a fast pace in answering questions is pointless if it makes you miss questions that you would have gotten right otherwise. Test writers like to include distracting information and wrong answers that seem right. Taking a little extra time to avoid careless mistakes can make all the difference in your test score. Find a pace that allows you to be confident in the answers that you select.

⊘ Keep Moving

Panicking will not help you pass the test, so do your best to stay calm and keep moving. Taking deep breaths and going through the answer elimination steps you practiced can help to break through a stress barrier and keep your pace.

Final Notes

The combination of a solid foundation of content knowledge and the confidence that comes from practicing your plan for applying that knowledge is the key to maximizing your performance on test day. As your foundation of content knowledge is built up and strengthened, you'll find that the strategies included in this chapter become more and more effective in helping you quickly sift through the distractions and traps of the test to isolate the correct answer.

Now that you're preparing to move forward into the test content chapters of this book, be sure to keep your goal in mind. As you read, think about how you will be able to apply this information on the test. If you've already seen sample questions for the test and you have an idea of the question format and style, try to come up with questions of your own that you can answer based on what you're reading. This will give you valuable practice applying your knowledge in the same ways you can expect to on test day.

Good luck and good studying!

14

General Laboratory

POLYPROPYLENE

Polypropylene is a type of plastic. Polypropylene is rigid, translucent, and it has a non-wettable surface, similar to Teflon. Polypropylene can also be autoclaved, because it has a melting point of 320 degrees Fahrenheit (160 degrees Celsius). This high melting point makes polypropylene able to withstand the high temperatures of an autoclave. In the laboratory, most pipette tips are made out of polypropylene, as are some test tubes and diluent trays.

POLYCARBONATE

Polycarbonate is another type of plastic. Sometimes, polycarbonate goes by the trademark name, Nalgene. Polycarbonate plastics are flexible, lightweight, and strong. They are able to withstand high impacts without breaking upon impact. In the laboratory, they can be used as a substitute for glass, because of their shatter-resistant capabilities.

POLYVINYLCHLORIDE (PVC)

Polyvinylchloride, or PVC, is a type of plastic. Polyvinylchloride is clear, can either be flexible or rigid, and it can also be either non-autoclavable or autoclavable. Flexible, autoclavable polyvinylchloride is used to make plastic tubing for use in the laboratory. This tubing can be used in various pieces of automated laboratory equipment, including continuous flow analyzers. Polyvinylchloride that is rigid and non-autoclavable is used to make plastic bottles for laboratory use.

POLYTETRAFLUOROETHYLENE

Polytetrafluoroethylene is a compound that sometimes goes by its trademark, Teflon. Teflon is a compound that has a slippery surface, and it is tough and stable over a wide range of temperatures It also has a non-wettable surface. In the laboratory, Teflon is used to make transfer disks for centrifugal analyzers, and it is also used to make stoppers and gaskets.

KIMAX GLASS

Kimax is a brand name for borosilicate glass. Borosilicate glasses contain at least 5% boric acid in their composition. They are also made up of sodium oxide, potassium oxide, calcium oxide, and silica. Borosilicate glasses are very heat resistant and strong as well. They also have a low thermal expansion coefficient, meaning that they do not expand much when heated. In the laboratory, flasks, beakers, and pipettes are usually made of borosilicate glass. Pyrex is another brand name of borosilicate glass products.

COREX GLASS

Corex is a brand name for aluminum-silicate glass. Aluminum-silicate glass is even stronger than borosilicate glass -- about six times stronger. Aluminum silicate glass also exhibits resistance to scratching and etching from alkaline materials. Corex glass is used in the laboratory in the form of thermometers and centrifuge tubes.

DESICCANTS USED IN THE LABORATORY

A desiccant is a material that readily absorbs water (hygroscopic). Desiccants are used to keep things dry and to prevent them from becoming hydrated or in contact with water. In the laboratory, some things that desiccants are used to keep dry are reagents, gases used in gas chromatography, and thin-layer chromatography (TLC) plates. Usually, a desiccator is used. A desiccator is typically

15

made out of glass, and the material in question is placed on a small shelf, with the desiccant placed below the shelf. A glass lid makes an air tight seal on the vessel. Some of the materials that can be used as desiccants include silica gel, calcium sulfate, sodium hydroxide, and magnesium perchloride. One of the least effective desiccants is silica gel, and the most effective desiccant is magnesium perchloride.

UNIVERSAL PRECAUTIONS

Universal precautions are used in the laboratory and other medical settings to help protect healthcare workers from diseases and poisons transmitted via bodily fluids and secretions (blood, semen, amniotic fluid, vaginal secretions, sweat, tears, saliva, urine, feces, wound drainage and CSF). Universal precautions became required practice after the outbreak of AIDS in 1980. Universal precautions means washing thoroughly and wearing protective gear, such as gloves, goggles or glasses, face shields, shoe covers, gowns, and anything else deemed appropriate by Infection Control. Which precautions need to be practiced in a given situation depend on the possibility of a healthcare worker coming in contact with the bodily fluids or secretions, not on the patient's known health status. Assume all patients are always infectious.

WORLD HEALTH ORGANIZATION (WHO) RULES

Each laboratory must have a manual that contains safety regulations. Labs should have sufficient workspace and accommodate disabled workers. Areas with patient access should be separate from the work area. The WHO has established rules for **laboratory safety**:

- The laboratory must be separate from areas of unrestricted traffic flow.
- Entry to the laboratory should be through double doors or a vestibule.
- All surfaces should be water-resistant for easy cleaning and well sealed, impervious to water, and resistant to chemicals, such as acids and solvents.
- The laboratory itself must be sealable and allow for gaseous decontamination.
- Windows must be kept closed and sealed, and must be resistant to breakage.
- Airflow must be into the laboratory from access rooms.
- Negative pressure airflow must be maintained and intake and output filtered through a HEPA filter. Output must be discharged outside of the building and at a distance from air intakes.
- The water supply must be outfitted with anti-backflow devices.
- All effluent must be decontaminated before discharged into the sewer system.
- Biological safety cabinets must have a negative airflow filter.

EQUIPMENT SAFETY

Equipment safety is essential because lancets, needles, and other sharp objects pose risks to laboratory personnel and must be used properly and disposed of safely in specific ("sharps") containers designed for safety. Procedures should be in place for all use of sharps and standard precautions followed. Safety lancets with needles that automatically retract should be utilized if possible. Safety needles are also available; if using a standard needle, the needle should not be recapped or bent prior to disposal but placed directly into the container, sharp end downward. Sharps containers should be leak-proof, resistant to punctures, clearly labeled, and placed in a convenient place not accessible by children. Most sharps containers are red, but clear containers may also be used so it is easier to see when they are full. Containers should never be filled to the top because of the risk that a needle or other sharp item may protrude through the opening.

16

PROPER STORAGE OF CHEMICALS IN THE LABORATORY

Proper storage of chemicals in the laboratory is vital to maintaining technician safety and a safe work place. All lab chemicals must have the proper labels and be stored in the proper container. For example, materials that are flammable need to be stored in a fire safety cabinet, to minimize the risk of fire. Solvents, on the other hand, need to be stored in a refrigerator that is explosion-proof. In addition to using proper storage containers and equipment, chemicals that are incompatible with each other should never be stored together. An example of this would be storing oxidizing agents next to reducing agents. Therefore, chemicals should never be stored alphabetically, as this may place incompatible chemicals next to each other in a storage situation. The amount of flammable substances and solvents that are stored should be limited, further reducing the risk of fire. Store large containers on a low shelf, close to the ground, to minimize dangers if these containers break. Check storage areas monthly to make sure that everything is stored properly.

COLLECTING BLOOD SAMPLES

Safety precautions when collecting blood samples include:

1. Plan ahead and ensure all needed supplies are on hand.
2. Wear a lab coat that is fully buttoned to protect clothing.
3. Carry out proper hand hygiene before and after procedures.
4. Wear gloves for phlebotomy procedures and any processing.
5. Follow standard precautions throughout the procedure.
6. Utilize safety-engineered devices, such as retractable needles and lancets, and single-use devices when possible.
7. Do not recap or bend needles prior to disposal.
8. If recapping of a needle is necessary, use one-hand scooping method.
9. Dispose of needles and syringes as one unit rather than separating.
10. Dispose of sharps in appropriate containers.
11. Ensure immunization for hepatitis B is current.
12. Immediately report any exposure to blood or body fluids and begin PEP if needed.
13. Ensure the work area for collection is well lighted and clean.
14. Follow protocols for blood collection.
15. Obtain assistance for unruly or confused patients.
16. Place sample tube in rack prior to injecting sample through rubber stopper.

INFECTION CONTROL

Each laboratory should carry out a biological risk assessment each year or when new risks arise to determine the biosafety level and agent hazards and procedures hazards. Work practices should conform to Bloodborne Pathogen Standard (Occupational Safety and Health Administration [OSHA]) and standard precautions (CDC). **Infection control** precautions include:

1. Utilizing appropriate hand hygiene with hand-free sink for washing hands available near exit.
2. Using mechanical pipettes instead of mouth pipetting.
3. Eating, drinking, smoking, storing food, applying makeup, and handling contact lenses all prohibited in the laboratory.
4. Maintaining safe handling of sharps policies.
5. Utilizing safety devices (retractable needles, lances) when possible.
6. Minimizing splashing or aerosolizing liquids.
7. Decontaminating potentially infectious materials prior to disposal.

8. Packing potentially infectious materials for disposal outside of facility in appropriate packaging according to regulations.
9. Maintaining a pest management program.
10. Ensuring that all personnel are adequately trained.
11. Ensuring appropriate immunizations and screening for personnel.
12. Making PPE available and monitoring appropriate use.
13. Ensuring eye wash station is easily accessed and available.

TYPES OF FIRE EXTINGUISHERS

1. Type A: fires caused by combustible materials, e.g. paper, plastic, wood, rubber, and cloth
2. Type B: fires caused by flammable liquids, e.g. paint thinner, grease, and oil
3. Type C: fires of electrical origin
4. Type D: fires caused by combustible metals, as for instance potassium, magnesium, titanium, sodium, and lithium
5. Multipurpose: fires caused by combustible metals, combustible materials, or flammable liquids; i.e., Type A, B, and C fires

CLEANING UP CHEMICAL SPILLS IN THE LABORATORY

1. Solvent spills: activated charcoal should be placed around the perimeter of the spill and then mixed in with the solvent; once it is possible, the mixture of activated charcoal and solvent should be swept into a plastic bag; protective glasses and gloves should be worn at all times
2. Acid spills: acid neutralizer, as for instance sodium bicarbonate, should be placed around the perimeter; neutralizer should be mixed with acid until it is safe to wipe the mixture into a plastic bag; bag should then be put into a fume hood; protective glasses and gloves should be worn at all times

REAGENT GRADE WATER

Reagent grade water is either type I, type II, or type III. Type III reagent grade water is only used to rinse glassware in the laboratory. Type II reagent grade water can be used for basic laboratory practices, it can only be stored for a brief period of time before it is subject to contamination. Type I reagent grade water is of the highest quality and is used in those cases when precision is most important. These three types of water are typically prepared using the following methods: reverse osmosis, activated carbon filters, sub micron filters, glass pre-filters, and cotton pre-filters.

CLSI QUALITY CONTROL PROCEDURES

The **Clinical and Laboratory Standards Institute** (CLSI) provides standards for a wide range of performance and testing and cover all types of laboratory functions and microbiology. These standards are used as a basis for quality control procedures. Standards include:

- Labeling: The label must be 2 inches × 1 inch and contain the required elements (patient name (left upper corner), unique identifier, birth date, date and time of collection, and collector's signature or ID.
- Security/Information technology: Technical operational and implementation requirements for *in vitro* analytical equipment and data management must be followed and essential elements included and de-identification practices utilized.
- Toxicology/Drug testing: Protocols for collecting, analyzing, interpreting, and reporting results of drug testing should be used as the basis for development of procedures.

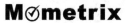

- Statistical quality control/Quantitative measurements: Provides guidance for quality control of different measurement procedures to ensure accuracy and safety of laboratory personnel.
- Performance standards for various types of antimicrobial susceptibility testing.

LABORATORY PROCEDURES AND ACCEPTANCE OR REJECTION OF AN ANALYSIS

As part of **quality control**, only personnel who are properly trained and qualified through education should be employed in the laboratory. Measures to ensure quality control include:

- Checking speed of centrifuge, volumes dispensed by diluters, temperature of water baths, and proper storage and expiration dates of reagents.
- Checking for proper instrument handling.
- Ensuring that appropriate organisms are used for sensitivity testing.
- Double-checking negative reports (especially in parasitology) by supervising personnel.
- Evaluating processing time to ensure samples are tested within the appropriate window, such as 2 hours for urine specimens and 4 hours for white blood cell counts.
- Correlating results, such as reviewing both hemoglobin and hematocrit.
- Maintaining accurate and appropriate records.
- Preparing a quality control chart.
- Establishing standards and controls for daily laboratory operation.
- Establishing standards and protocols for acceptance or rejection of samples and analysis.
- Applying Westgard's rule to determine acceptable variation in control before rejecting test results.
- Determining if a run has occurred to indicate results are out of control and should be rejected.

CLINICAL LABORATORY IMPROVEMENT AMENDMENTS (CLIA)

In the United States, all laboratory testing, except for research, is regulated by the CMS (Centers for Medicare and Medicaid Services) through **Clinical Laboratory Improvement Amendments (CLIA).** CLIA is implemented through the Division of Laboratory Services and serves approximately 244,000 laboratories. Laboratories receiving reimbursement from CMS must meet CLIA standards, which ensure that laboratory testing will be accurate and procedures followed properly. The Centers for Disease Control and Prevention (CDC) partners with CMS and the Food and Drug Administration (FDA) in supporting CLIA programs. Physician office laboratories are most often accredited by COLA (Commission on Laboratory Accreditation), founded in 1988 with the original intent of inspecting and accrediting physician office laboratories to ensure that they were in compliance with CLIA. COLA has since expanded its mission and now also accredits hospital laboratories as well as independent laboratories. CMS and the Joint Commission have granted deeming authority to COLA.

PROFICIENCY TESTING

Proficiency testing is a method of quality control that assesses the performance (accuracy and reliability) of a laboratory in carrying out tests and measurements, comparing laboratory results with those of other laboratories. Samples that have been previously tested by reference laboratories to establish reference values are sent to the laboratory by a CMS-approved proficiency testing agency for blind testing and the results are checked against those obtained by the reference laboratories. Samples are generally sent to participating laboratories about every 4 months with 5 samples sent each time with at least 1 sample specific to the type of testing the lab carries out, such as gram stains and organism identification. Testing must be carried out on the samples in the same manner as actual patient specimens, and samples may not be forwarded to other laboratories for testing or to verify results. The results are submitted to the proficiency testing agency, which grades the findings and sends the laboratory a score. Both CMS and accreditation agencies routinely monitor these scores.

QUALITY IMPROVEMENT
TOTAL QUALITY MANAGEMENT (TQM)

Total Quality Management (TQM) is one philosophy of quality management that espouses a commitment to meeting the needs of the customers at all levels within an organization. It promotes not only continuous improvement but also a dedication to quality in all aspects of an organization. Outcomes should include increased customer satisfaction and productivity, as well as increased profits through efficiency and reduction in costs. In order to provide TQM, an organization must seek the following:

- Information regarding customer's needs and opinions.
- Involvement of staff at all levels in decision making, goal setting, and problems solving.
- Commitment of management to empowering staff and being accountable through active leadership and participation.
- Institution of teamwork with incentives and rewards for accomplishments.
- The focus of TQM is on working together to identify and solve problems rather than assigning blame through an organizational culture that focuses on the needs of the customers.

CONTINUOUS QUALITY IMPROVEMENT (CQI)

Continuous Quality Improvement (CQI) emphasizes the organization and systems and processes within that organization rather than individuals. It recognizes internal customers (staff) and external customers (patients) and utilizes data to improve processes. CQI represents the concept that most processes can be improved. CQI uses the scientific method of experimentation to meet needs and improve services and utilizes various tools, such as brainstorming, multivoting, various charts and diagrams, storyboarding, and meetings. Core concepts include:

- Quality and success is meeting or exceeding internal and external customer's needs and expectations.
- Problems relate to processes, and variations in process lead to variations in results.
- Change can be in small steps.

Steps to CQI include:

- Forming a knowledgeable team.
- Identifying and defining measures used to determine success.
- Brainstorming strategies for change.
- Plan, collect, and utilize data as part of making decisions.
- Test changes and revise or refine as needed.

PERFORMANCE IMPROVEMENT COUNCIL (PIC)

The **Performance Improvement Council (PIC)** was developed by the US government (Title 31, Code 1124) as an interagency collaborative effort to share information in order to improve performance and management, although the principles of openness and sharing can also be applied to the private sector. Members of the PIC include performance improvement officers as well as representatives from various federal agencies and departments. These members of the central PIC

20

work together to facilitate communication and share best practices by providing consultation services and facilitators to help others develop cross-agency teams and establish priority goals. The PIC actively seeks information regarding best practices from both governmental and private sector entities. Each governmental agency must assign a performance improvement officer whose responsibility is to improve performance and coordinate with interagency councils. The PIC is active in setting goals as well as measurement and analysis, including performance review and capacity building.

PREANALYTICAL, ANALYTICAL, AND/OR POSTANALYTICAL CAUSES OF ERRONEOUS RESULTS

Erroneous results may occur because of problems in any step in the collection and processing of specimens, but the greatest danger of errors occurs in the preanalytical stage, where many different things can go wrong:

- Preanalytical errors: Include hemolysis of specimen, inappropriate request for test, error in order entry, inadequate sample volume/size, use of incorrect tube, improper identification of patient, improper preservation method for specimen, tube breakage (before or during centrifugation), inadequate centrifugation (time/speed), delayed transport, reagent expired, ID or barcode unclear, duplicate pathological numbers, and specimens mixed up.
- Analytical errors: Include quality control failure and malfunctioning of equipment resulting in improper results.
- Postanalytical errors: Include failure to post results, error in interpretation of results, excessive turnaround time, and failure to collect results.

ASSURING CONTINUAL ACCURACY OF PATIENT IDENTIFICATION IN ALL SITUATIONS

The first step in any blood draw or laboratory procedure for inpatients and outpatients should be to properly **identify the patient**, using at least 2 forms of identification. Alert and responsive patients (or parents of a minor) may be asked to give their names and birthdates:

- Check ID band against information provided by patient/caregiver/parent.
- Match specimen labeling to information on ID band and label immediately with barcode labeler or permanent ink.
- Check ankles for ID band if missing from wrists.
- Consider only ID bands actually on the patient as valid (not on bedside stand/bed) except in special circumstances (severe burns of extremities). Verify ID with nurse in these cases.
- If armband missing, procure armband and secure on patient before procedure.
- Ask outpatients for picture ID and verify name and birthdate verbally if possible.
- For emergent situations (unconscious patient in ED), check "Jane/John Doe" ID as per protocol.
- For call reports, verify patient's name, birthdate, and ID number.

QUALITY ASSURANCE MEASURES RELATED TO AUTOCLAVING

Quality assurance testing of an autoclave determines if an autoclave can reach a correct temperature for a long enough period of time, usually 121 degree Celsius for fifteen minutes. Striped tape and chemical indicators are used. A color change will indicate when the temperature and time conditions have been reached. Physical indicators, such as a melting metal alloy, can also indicate that the required conditions have been met. A biological indicator, a suspension containing spores of *Bacillus stearothermophilus*, can also be used. This particular bacterium is heat resistant, so if the required autoclave conditions have not been met, the spores will germinate, and deteriorate the glucose that is present in the suspension. Color changes from purple to yellow. However, if the autoclave conditions have been met, spores will not germinate, and there will be no viable spores visible after an incubation period of seven days at 55 degrees Celsius, and no color change.

MANUAL INSTRUMENTATION

Borosilicate glassware is heat and chemical resistant; soda lime glassware, less expensive and less resistant; and plastic ware, less expensive and less breakable but not heat resistant and cannot be used with some reagents and chemicals. Commonly used **manual laboratory instrumentation** includes:

1. Test tubes: Used to heat and hold reagents to assess chemical reactions. Vary in size and usually rimless. Held in plastic or metal test tube racks. Centrifuge tubes (15 mL) are similar but have tapered ends to hold pellet. Cuvettes are rectangular test tubes to hold solutions for photometry, placed only in plastic racks to avoid scratching.
2. Funnels (plain and separating): Supported in ring stand and used for filtration or to separate immiscible liquids.
3. General purpose and volumetric glassware: Includes graduated cylinders, volumetric flasks, pipettes, and burettes and used for measuring volumes. Pipettes or eyedroppers are used to transfer liquids. Mouth pipettes should never be used. Reagent bottles hold reagents. Beakers are used to heat liquids.

CLEANING AND MAINTENANCE OF MANUAL INSTRUMENTATION

Cleaning and maintenance of manual instrumentation: All glassware and plastic ware should be rinsed immediately after use in hot tap water to prevent substances from drying. The rinsed ware is soaked in low suds detergent solution (2%) for at least an hour. The ware is then scrubbed with appropriately-sized brushes inside and out. Chromic acid may be used to remove coagulated organic material. Each item is washed 5 times under running tap water to remove all detergent followed by 3 rinses with distilled or deionized water. After the washing and rinsing are completed, the equipment is dried in an oven at 140°C if heat resistant or placed in a drying rack overnight. Prior to first use of newly purchased glassware, items made of borosilicate glass should be cleaned with detergent, washed under tap water, and rinsed with distilled/deionized water. Items made of soda lime glass should be soaked overnight in 5% hydrochloric acid, diluted 6 times to 30% to neutralize free alkali before washing under tap water, and rinsed with distilled/deionized water.

ADVANTAGES AND DISADVANTAGES OF AUTOMATED LABORATORY INSTRUMENTATION

Automated laboratory instrumentation is becoming the norm, and a laboratory may have total laboratory automation or system-based automation. Automated laboratory instrumentation has a number of advantages over manual procedures:

- Test results can be obtained faster and are often more accurate because they are not dependent on varying techniques and subjective judgment.
- Test results are more reliable and consistent, and can be easily reproduced.
- Data can be more easily stored, transferred, manipulated, and reported.
- Fewer laboratory personnel are needed because the automated systems can do the work of many technicians.
- Errors are minimized.
- Workflow is more efficient.

However, there are also some disadvantages: If a machine breaks down, there may be considerable delay in manually producing lab reports because of inadequate staffing or equipment. Additionally, staff members must be trained in trouble shooting and maintenance of equipment and service technicians must be available. The automation equipment may be prohibitively expensive, especially for a small laboratory.

CALIBRATION OF INSTRUMENTS

Generally, all instruments used to generate, measure, and assess data should be routinely calibrated and tested, based on standards and standard operating procedures. The frequency may vary, but some require daily **calibration** while others need calibration every few months. Equipment should also be calibrated if mechanical or other problems have occurred. Calibration may be done manually or semi- or completely automatically, and procedures may vary, but usually include:

1. Testing calibrators, solutions, or samples with known values, to determine accuracy of measurement.
2. Carefully preparing calibrators, including correct volumes.
3. Following directions exactly (according to manufacturer's guidelines), maintaining the proper conditions (light, heat, ventilation), and using calibrators in the correct order and manner.
4. Noting the need for adjustments to the equipment or process.

Calibration is part of quality control, but those instruments, supplies, or equipment that are not involved in directly generating, measuring, or assessing data generally do not require calibration but are maintained as part of general quality control.

SETTING UP, BALANCING, AND OPERATING A CENTRIFUGE

Centrifuges spin solutions to separate out solid materials by forcing them away from the center to form a pellet. Centrifuges come in various sizes and may be free floating/horizontal or angle-head (45-degree angle). Different specimens require different G-forces/relative centrifugal force (RCF) (which is the spinning force relative to earth's gravitation) and different durations. The G-force/RCF depends on the revolutions per minute (RPMs) and the radius of revolution (RR) (measured in mm from the center to the end of the test tube): RCF/G-force = $1.12 \times RR \times (RPM/1000)^2$ (or use nomogram chart). Procedure:

1. Use equal numbers of tubes in the buckets on opposite sites. Weigh tubes to ensure the load is balanced and use a tube filled with water if testing an odd number.
2. Close and lock centrifuge, turn it on, and follow instructions for settings.
3. Spin for necessary duration (such as 15 to 20 minutes). If excessive vibration (from imbalance) or sound of cracking vial occurs, turn off machine.
4. When completed, remove buckets carefully to avoid jarring the pellets.
5. Open buckets and remove tubes, checking for sediments.

MICROSCOPY

The **microscope** most commonly used is the <u>light microscope</u> (either monocular or binocular). This microscope uses external light or light from an internal filament that allows the light to pass upward through the specimen so that the specimen appears dark against the lighter background, although the light may be inverted, illuminating from the top, for such things as a culture in a liquid medium. <u>Phase contrast microscopes</u> that do not require staining of the specimen are used to assess cell growth, especially for organisms that are transparent with standard light microscope. The <u>dark field microscope</u> uses a special dark-field condenser that makes the specimen appear light against a dark background, useful for observing spirochetes. The <u>fluorescent microscope</u> utilizes an ultraviolet light for illumination. This microscope is used when fluorescent dye is attached to a specimen because the dye glows when exposed to ultraviolet light, useful for fluorescent antibody testing.

CALIBRATION OF AN OCULAR MICROMETER

The ocular micrometer is a glass disk that fits into the microscope eyepiece and provides an engraved ruler for measurement within the ocular lens. The **ocular micrometer calibration** procedure is as follows:

- Remove eyepiece and unscrew the ocular eye lens and position the ocular micrometer with the engraved ruler with 100 divisions face down, replace the lens, and place the ocular with the micrometer into the ocular tube and microscope with 10× objective.
- Place a stage micrometer slide with an engraved scale that closely matches in the ocular micrometer length and number of divisions on the microscope stage and focus on the parallel sets of rulers so that the 0-mm lines on the ocular micrometer and stage micrometer align.
- Locate another set of lines that align at the furthest distance from the 0-mm lines.
- Count the number of lines between the 0-mm alignment and the distant alignment on both the ocular micrometer scale and the stage micrometer scale.
- Use formulas to determine the proportion of a mm measured by 1 ocular unit:
- Stage micrometer reading × 1000 micrometers/ocular micrometer reading × 1 mm = ocular units.
- For 40× objective: 0.1 mm × 1000 micrometer/50 units × 1 mm.

HARDWARE

Computer hardware consists of all of the physical parts of a computer. All machinery and equipment that makes up the computer and its related components are considered hardware. This includes computer disks, cables, the CPU (central processing unit), printers, keyboard, modem, and any other physical parts of the computer. A computer's hardware is what indicates what a computer is capable of doing.

SOFTWARE

Computer software, on the other hand, is all of the programs that tell a computer how to operate. Software can be divided into application software, which are programs that manipulate and process data, and system software, which control the computer and other programs. Software is written in various programming languages, and the software is responsible for controlling what the hardware does and how the hardware operates.

BENEFIT OF COMPUTERIZED DATA AUTOMATION IN THE LABORATORY

Computerized automation of laboratory data has several advantages. For one, with the computer taking care of recording and storing data, laboratory technicians have more time to do other clinical tasks, such as performing laboratory tests. This increases laboratory productivity. Data stored on a computer, instead of paper laboratory reports, requires less storage space and can be encrypted for confidentiality. Another reason that computer automation is beneficial is that with data stored in a computer system, doctors and nurses can access such data much faster than if paper reports had to be mailed or faxed to them. In some cases, doctors can log onto a hospital computer system to see test results right away. And, using a computer to record data leads to fewer filing and billing errors on the part of the laboratory technicians.

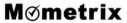

ORDERING SETS OF DATA MEASUREMENTS EXAMPLES

The following conversions are helpful for this problem: 1 character = 1 byte; 1 byte = 8 bits; 1 Kbyte = 1024 bytes.

Order the following set of data measurements measurements in order of lowest to highest memory:

5 characters, 1 Kbyte, 20 bytes, 16,000 bits

In this situation, it would be helpful to convert everything to one common unit, such as bytes. So, 5 characters = 5 bytes; 1 Kbyte = 1024 bytes; 16,000 bits = 2000 bytes. 20 bytes does not need to be converted. Therefore, in order from lowest to highest memory, the order is: 5 characters, 20 bytes, 1Kbyte, 16,000 bits.

Order the following set of data measurements measurements in order of lowest to highest memory:

24,000 bits, 1000 characters, 500 bytes, 4 Kbyte

In this situation, it would be helpful again to convert everything to one common unit, such as bytes. So, 24,000 bits = 3000 bytes; 1000 characters = 1000 bytes; 4 Kbyte = 4096 bytes. 500 bytes does not need to be converted. Therefore, in order from lowest to highest memory, the order is: 500 bytes, 1000 characters, 24,000 bits, 4 Kbyte.

APPROPRIATE METHODS TO MAINTAIN THE SECURITY OF LABORATORY COMPUTERS AND DATABASES

Security of laboratory computers and databases is a very important issue in the medical laboratory. Patient confidentiality must be kept at all times, and patients' data must not get into the wrong hands or be viewed by the wrong set of eyes. Because of this, there are various methods that laboratories can use to keep their computers and databases safe. Using passwords and identification numbers or names for each laboratory technician or doctor is a widely used method for security. Also, limiting the access to the computers can help as well. Using voice recognition technologies or keys that must be inserted into locks on the computers can keep computers and data safe. Various software programs, such as anti-virus, anti-spyware, and encryption software can enhance security. It must be noted, however, that security measures should not greatly impact the ease of using the computers.

EXAMPLE MOLARITY PROBLEM

Determine the molarity (M) of a solution that contains 20.0 grams of NaCl in 500 mL of solution.

The molarity (M) of a solution is equal to moles per liter. In this example, we need to calculate what one mole (gram molecular weight) is of NaCl first. A mole of a compound is equal to the sum of the atomic weights of the elements in that compound. So, for NaCl, one mole is equal to the atomic weight of Na plus the atomic weight of Cl (23.0g + 35.5g), or 58.5 g. Next, it is best to determine the concentration of the solution in terms of grams per liter. So, in our example, the solution is 20.0 g NaCl/500 mL. This is equivalent to 20.0g NaCl/0.5 L, or 40g NaCl/L. Next, the number of moles of NaCl present in the solution must be calculated. Take the grams of NaCl present in 1 liter of solution and divide it by the weight of one mole of NaCl (40g NaCl/58.5g NaCl). In our example, the number of moles present is therefore equal to 0.68 moles. Since molarity is equal to moles per liter, the molarity of this solution is therefore 0.68 mol/L, or the solution is a 0.68 M NaCl solution.

SAMPLE CONVERSION PROBLEMS

Convert 55 degrees Fahrenheit to degrees Celsius.

To convert from degrees Fahrenheit to degrees Celsius, the following equation is used: degrees Celsius = (degrees Fahrenheit - 32) x 5/9. Plugging in the number given for degrees Fahrenheit, 55, the degrees Celsius is calculated to be approximately 13 degrees.

Convert 32 degrees Fahrenheit to degrees Celsius.

To convert from degrees Fahrenheit to degrees Celsius, the following equation is used: degrees Celsius = (degrees Fahrenheit – 32) x 5/9. Using the number given for degrees Fahrenheit, 32, the degrees Celsius is calculated to be 0 degrees.

Convert 12 degrees Celsius to degrees Fahrenheit.

To convert from degrees Celsius to degrees Fahrenheit, the following equation is used: degrees Fahrenheit = (degrees Celsius x 9/5) + 32. Plugging in the number given for degrees Celsius, 12, the degrees Fahrenheit is calculated to be approximately 54 degrees.

Convert 31 degrees Celsius to degrees Fahrenheit.

To convert from degrees Celsius to degrees Fahrenheit, the following equation is used: degrees Fahrenheit = (degrees Celsius x 9/5) + 32. Plugging in the number given for degrees Celsius, 31, the degrees Fahrenheit is calculated to be approximately 88 degrees.

BEER'S LAW

Beer's law is defined as A = abc, where A is the absorbance, a is the absorptivity, b is the path of light in centimeters (cm), and c is the concentration of the absorbing compound.

EXAMPLE BEER'S LAW CALCULATION PROBLEM

For a certain spectrophotometric procedure, the absorbance of a standard solution (concentration is 25 mg/dL) is 0.75 (in a 1 cm cell). The absorbance of the sample solution is 0.35 (in a 1 cm cell). Calculate the concentration of the sample solution.

For the problem given, both b (the path of light in centimeters) and a (the absorptivity) are constant. So, using Beer's law, the equation then becomes: $c_{sample}/c_{standard} = A_{sample}/A_{standard}$. All of the values in that equation are known except for the concentration of the sample, c_{sample}. Rearranging the equation gives: $c_{sample} = A_{sample}/A_{standard} \times c_{standard}$. Plugging in the values given in the problem gives the following: $c_{sample} = 0.35/0.75 \times 25$ mg/dL or 11.7 mg/dL. 11.7 mg/dL is the concentration of the sample solution.

OSMOLALITY

Osmolality is defined as the moles per 1 kilogram (kg) of solvent multiplied by the number of particles into which the molecules of solute dissociate.

EXAMPLE OSMOLALITY CALCULATION PROBLEMS

Calculate the osmolality of 54 g glucose and 11.7 g NaCl in 2 kg of water.

To calculate the osmolality in the given problem, first we need to calculate how many moles of solute (both glucose and NaCl) are present. For glucose, 54 g of glucose = 54 g/180 g/mol = 0.3 mol glucose. For NaCl, 11.7 g NaCl = 11.7 g/58.5 g/mol = 0.2 mol NaCl. Then, we need to look at how each solute dissociates. Glucose does not really dissociate well. However, 0.2 mol of NaCl will dissociate into two particles, 0.2 mol of Na^+ and 0.2 mol of Cl^-. So, to calculate the number of Osmoles present, we would add 0.3 Osmole of glucose to 0.2 Osmole of Na^+ and 0.2 Osmole of Cl^-. This totals 0.7 Osmoles present. Because we are dealing with 2 kg of water, however, and osmolality is noted as moles per 1 kilogram, we need to divide 0.7 Osmoles by 2 kg of water, to give 0.35 Osmoles per 1 kg of water, or 0.35 Osmolal.

Determine how many grams of NaCl are required to prepare 250 mL of a 3 M solution.

1 *M* solution (or 1 molar solution) is equal to 1 mole of solution divided by 1 liter of solution. So, for this problem, first, the molecular weight of 1 mole of NaCl must be calculated. That value is 58.5 g. Therefore, 1 liter of a 1 *M* solution of NaCl contains 58.5 grams. However, since we are interested in a 3 *M* solution, the number of grams contained in a 1 *M* solution must be multiplied by 3. Therefore, a 3 *M* solution contains 3 x 58.5 g/L, or 175.5 g/L. In this problem, though, only 250 g of the 3 *M* solution are needed. So, the 3 *M* solution needs to be multiplied by the volume needed. This equation then becomes: 175.5 g/L x 250 mL/1000mL, or 43.9 g NaCl. Therefore, in order to prepare 250 mL of a 3 *M* solution of NaCl, 43.9 g of NaCl are needed.

DETERMINING FINAL CONCENTRATIONS OF SOLUTIONS EXAMPLES

Determine the final concentration, in normality (N), in the following situation:

A 2 *N* solution diluted 2:5 and then diluted 1:4

When calculating a final concentration of a solution after multiple dilutions, the initial concentration of the solution is multiplied by each of the dilutions (as a fraction). Therefore, to calculate the final concentration of this 2 *N* solution after being diluted 2:5 and 1:4, the equation used would be 2 *N* x 2/5 x ¼. The final concentration would then be 0.2 *N*.

Determine the final concentration, in normality (N), in the following situation:

A 5 *N* solution diluted 1:2, then diluted 2:3, and then diluted 3:5

In this situation, the equation used to calculate the final concentration of the solution after undergoing multiple dilutions as stated would be: 5 *N* x ½ x 2/3 x 3/5. The final concentration of this solution is then calculated to be 1 *N*.

Determine the final concentration, in normality (N), in the following situation:

A 4 *N* solution diluted 3:7, then diluted 6:13, and then diluted 1:2

In this particular situation, the equation used to calculate the final concentration of the solution after undergoing three separate dilutions as stated in the problem

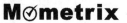

would be: 4 *N* x 3/7 x 6/13 x ½. Using this equation, the final concentration of the solution can be calculated to be 0.4 *N*.

CALCULATING THE CONCENTRATION IN MILLIEQUIVALENTS PER LITER (mEq/L) EXAMPLES

Calculate the concentration in milliequivalents per liter (mEq/L) of the following:

serum potassium level of 22.3 mg/dL

To calculate a concentration in milliequivalents per liter (mEq/L), when given concentration in milligrams per deciliter (mg/dL), the following equation needs to be used: (mg/dL x 10 dL/L x valence) / atomic mass = mEq/L. So, for potassium, the valence of potassium is 1, and the atomic mass of potassium is 39. These values can be obtained by using a periodic table. Therefore, the equation then becomes (22.3 mg/dL x 10 dL/L x 1) / 39 = 5.7 mEq/L.

Calculate the concentration in milliequivalents per liter (mEq/L) of the following:

serum calcium level of 9.0 mg/dL

For this example, we can use the same equation as in part a to calculate mEq/L; (mg/dL x 10 dL/L x valence) / atomic mass = mEq/L. For calcium, the valence is 2, and the atomic mass is 40. Therefore, the equation then becomes (9.0 mg/dL x 10 dL/L x 2) / 40 = 4.5 mEq/L.

TASK ANALYSIS

Task analysis involves breaking down all of the specific points or elements that are involved in performing a specific task. This can involve all of the skills or knowledge that are needed, the time involved, the equipment needed to perform the task, among other things.

OBJECTIVES

An objective is a statement that tells one what they should be able to do/know/understand after completing a course of instruction. An objective will describe specific behaviors or knowledge that should be learned.

GOALS

A goal is similar to an objective, except that it is more generalized. It does not discuss specific behaviors or pieces of knowledge, but it discusses what one should be able to do after completing a course of instruction in the general sense.

COURSE DESCRIPTIONS

A course description describes the content of the course the description is associated with. Unlike goals or objectives, what the student is supposed to learn (whether specific as in an objective or general as in a goal) is not part of a course description.

MAJOR DOMAINS FOR BEHAVIORAL OBJECTIVES

The three major domains for behavioral objectives are cognitive, affective, and psychomotor. The cognitive domain deals with objectives related to the intellect and learning. This includes memory, thinking, reasoning, analysis, language, synthesis, and evaluation, among other aspects. The affective domain deals more with attitudes, values, and emotions. The affective domain is essentially the opposite of the cognitive or thinking domain. Some behaviors that the affective domain includes are lab safety procedures and techniques, and patient confidentiality. Finally, the

28

psychomotor domain includes objectives related to actually performing a task or doing something physically. The performance of laboratory procedures would fall under the psychomotor domain of behavioral objectives.

CALCULATING THE DISCRIMINATION INDEX EXAMPLE

Calculate the discrimination index for a particular test question associated with the following information: number of students in the lower 27% group is 17; number of students in the upper 27% group is 17; number of students in the lower group answering this test question correctly is 6; number of students in the higher group answering this test question correctly is 14.

The discrimination index is calculated by subtracting the number of students in the lower group answering correctly from the number of students in the upper group answering correctly, and dividing that result by the number of students in either the upper or the lower group. The number of students in the lower group and the number of students in the upper group are based on test scores, with 27% of the test takers falling into each the lower and the upper group. For this problem, this equation used to calculate discrimination index would be (14-6) / 17, or 8 / 17, or .47 Therefore, the discrimination index for this particular test question is 0.47. The discrimination index can be any number between + 1.0 and – 1.0. Discrimination indices over 0.4 are desired.

DETERMINING THE PAID PRODUCTIVITY EXAMPLE

Determine the paid productivity in the following situation, with the following conditions: three full time equivalents work in the laboratory; each employee gets paid for 2200 hours annually; each full time equivalent actually works 2000 hours annually; the three full time equivalents together produce 285,000 work load units annually.

Paid productivity is equal to the total number of work load units divided by the total paid hours per year. In this situation, the number of work load units (WLUs) is equal to 285,000. The total paid hours per year is the number of hours each full time equivalent gets paid for each year multiplied by the number of full time equivalents (FTEs). In this situation, the total paid hours per year is equal to 2200 hours multiplied by 3 full time equivalents, or 6600. So, to calculate paid productivity, the number of work load units (285,000) is divided by the total paid hours per year (6600). This gives a value of 43.18 work load units paid per hour. To calculate the paid productivity as a percentage, divide the work load units paid per hour (43.18) by 60 minutes (because there are 60 minutes in an hour), and multiply by 100. This gives a paid productivity of 71.97%.

DETERMINING WORKED PRODUCTIVITY EXAMPLE

Determine the worked productivity in the following situation, with the following conditions: three full time equivalents work in the laboratory; each employee gets paid for 2200 hours annually; each full time equivalent actually works 2000 hours annually; the three full time equivalents together produce 285,000 work load units annually.

Worked productivity is equal to the total number of work load units divided by the total number of hours worked per year. In this situation, the number of work load units (WLUs) is equal to 285,000. The total number of hours worked per year is equal to the number of hours each full time equivalent actually works per year multiplied by the number of full time equivalents (FTEs). In this situation, the total number of hours worked per year is equal to 2000 hours multiplied by 3 full time equivalents, or 6000. So, to calculate worked productivity, the number of work load units (285,000) is divided by the total number of hours worked per year (6000). This gives a value of 47.5 work load units per hour worked. To calculate the worked productivity as a percentage, divide the work load units per hour worked (47.5) by 60 minutes (because there are 60 minutes in an hour) and multiply by 100. This gives a worked productivity of 79.17%.

DETERMINING THE BREAKEVEN POINT FOR A NEW TEST EXAMPLE

Determine the breakeven point for a new test being used in the laboratory, noting the following conditions: revenue per unit is $12.00; fixed cost is $540.00; variable cost is $3.00. Also, net income in this situation is expected to be zero.

To calculate the break even point, the equation used is $rx = vx + f + c$. In this equation, x is the break even point, r is the revenue per unit, v is the variable cost, f is the fixed cost, and c is the net income. Plugging in the values given (note that net income is zero), the equation becomes $12x = 3x + 540 + 0$. Rearranging the equation to get the break even point (x) on one side of the equation, the equation becomes $12x - 3x = 540$, or $9x = 540$. Solving for x gives 60. This means that the break even point is 60. In other words, a minimum of 60 tests of this particular test must be performed in the laboratory for the laboratory to meet the break even point, with a net income of zero (no profit or no loss).

BLOOD, PLASMA, AND SERUM

Whole blood is blood as it is withdrawn from the body and contains plasma, which includes clotting factors; erythrocytes (red blood cells); leukocytes (white blood cells), which include monocytes, lymphocytes, neutrophils, basophils, and eosinophils; and thrombocytes (platelets). Whole blood is rarely used for testing or administration but is separated into components. **Plasma** is the liquid portion of the blood that is free of cells because the erythrocytes, leukocytes, and thrombocytes have been removed, but it still contains clotting factors, such as fibrinogen, because it has been treated with an anticoagulant, such as sodium citrate. **Serum**, on the other hand, is the liquid portion of blood that is cell free but has been allowed to clot and then spun to separate and remove the clot so that it is also free of clotting factors. Serum is more often used for testing than plasma because serum contains more antigens and can be used for a wider variety of tests. Additionally, anticoagulants found in plasma may interfere with some tests.

PREVENTING HEMOLYSIS

Hemolysis, rupture of red blood cells, is the most common reason laboratory specimens must be redrawn. Steps to preventing hemolysis include:

1. Utilize large gauge (20 to 22) needle for blood draws for large veins, such as the antecubital.
2. Warm draw site to improve blood flow.
3. Keep tourniquet on no longer than 60 seconds.
4. Air-dry alcohol applied to skin prior to blood draw.
5. Utilize partial vacuum tubes if possible.
6. Avoid milking veins or capillary puncture sites.
7. Avoid excessive pressure when pulling or pushing on plunger.
8. Avoid blood draws from catheters or vascular access devices.
9. Ensure volume in tubes with anticoagulant is sufficient.
10. Avoid vigorous mixing or shaking of specimens.

11. Invert tubes with clot activator 5 times, with anticoagulant 8 to 10 times, and with sodium citrate 3 to 4 times (coagulation tests).
12. Store and transport specimens at appropriate temperature.
13. Use appropriate centrifugal speed and duration for processing samples that have clotted completely.

COLLECTING BLOOD IN COLLECTING TUBES FOR ANALYSIS

Blood collection procedure:

1. Review order, obtain proper collection tubes and equipment.
2. Explain procedure to patient and obtain 2 forms of identification (such as name and birthdate).
3. Use correct hand hygiene according to protocol.
4. Position tourniquet 3 to 4 inches above draw site (typically antecubital area) and ask patient to make a fist.
5. Identify vein, release tourniquet, and have patient open fist.
6. Apply antiseptic and air dry.
7. Prepare equipment and don gloves.
8. Apply tourniquet again and ask patient to make a fist.
9. Anchor vein and carry out blood draw.
10. Release tourniquet and have patient open fist.
11. Place a tube in the holder and twist clockwise to make sure needle pierces the stopper.
12. Fill tubes according to order of the draw to avoid cross contamination of additives: Sample in tubes with clot activators (light blue, plastic red, gold and red/gray caps) or no additives (plain red cap) are obtained before samples in tubes with anticoagulant (green [heparin], royal blue [EDTA], and lavender [EDTA]).

USING COLLECTION TUBES WITH PROPER ANTICOAGULANT FOR THE TYPE OF ANALYSIS

Different labs may establish protocols that vary, so the order of the draw and tubes that are employed should be consulted. Typical color-capped collection tubs and anticoagulants include:

Collection cap	Anticoagulant	Tests
Green or Tan	Sodium heparin or Lithium heparin	Plasma chemistry tests, electrolytes, and cytogenetic tests (green-top, sodium heparin only)
Lavender	K2 EDTA	CBC and individual CBC components, sickle cell test, ESR
Royal blue	Spray dried K2 EDTA	Hematology (whole blood), ABO testing, RH typing, and antibody screening, nutritional testing and tests for lead and trace metals
Gray	Sodium heparin or Sodium fluoride (Na2)	Trace element tests, toxicology, and nutritional testing
	EDTA or potassium oxalate	Glucose testing (potassium oxalate)
Pink	EDTA	Blood bank specimens
Light blue	Sodium citrate	Coagulation tests

EFFECTS OF IMPROPER ANTICOAGULANT USE

A number of different **anticoagulants** are used and are designed for a specific type of testing, so using the wrong anticoagulant may make testing impossible or inaccurate:

1. <u>EDTA</u> preserves cell morphology and prevents clumping of platelets and is used for whole blood tests. Spray-dried EDTA is best for hematology tests because liquid EDTA can dilute the sample. EDTA contains high potassium levels and can result in increased potassium results.
2. <u>Citrates</u> prevent coagulation and are used for coagulation tests by adding back calcium to initiate the clotting process. The anticoagulant-blood ratio must be 1:9 because an underfilled tube prolongs clotting time.
3. <u>Heparin</u> inhibits thrombin formation. Lithium heparin cannot be used to test lithium levels as it will alter the test results, and sodium heparin cannot be used for sodium or electrolyte panels because the sodium levels will be inaccurate.
4. <u>Potassium oxalate</u> coagulates calcium to prevent coagulation and is usually added to tubes containing an antiglycolytic agent for glucose testing.

CLOTTING TIME FOR BLOOD SAMPLES

Clotting time may vary according to environmental conditions and addition of clot activators. Clotting must be fully complete before a sample is placed in the centrifuge or latent formation of fibrin may clot serum. Complete clotting usually takes between 30 and 60 minutes at temperatures of 22° to 25°C (room temperature), although this time may be prolonged in samples with a high white blood cell count or in chilled samples. Clotting is also prolonged in samples of patients on anticoagulant therapy, such as heparin or warfarin. Clot activators may be added to a sample to decrease the time needed for clotting:

- Silica particles (found in serum separator tubes) and plastic red-topped tubes require 15 to 30 minutes.
- Thrombin tubes require about 5 minutes.

Note: 5 to 6 gentle inversions of tubes with clot activators to mix it with the blood sample are required.

BLOOD CULTURE COLLECTION PROCEDURE

Blood culture collection:

1. Verify patient identification with 2 identifiers.
2. Use standard precautions and venipuncture procedures, and use aseptic technique when handling equipment to avoid contamination.
3. Vigorously scrub skin with antiseptic for 30 to 60 seconds to remove skin bacteria and allow to dry.
4. Swab caps of blood culture bottles with antiseptic. Note fill line.
5. Carry out blood draw. Adults: 10-20 mL per set and pediatric patients 1-2 mL per set.
6. If multiple draws are ordered, wait 30 minutes between draws unless otherwise ordered. Take multiple draws from different sites.
7. Replace venipuncture needle with blunt fill needle and use transfer device.
8. Inject blood culture specimen into both anaerobic and aerobic bottles (anaerobic first if syringe used, but aerobic first if butterfly used because air from the tubing will enter the bottle), controlling flow so the entire volume is not sucked into the first bottle.
9. Mix specimen with medium in the culture bottle according to directions.

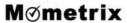

10. Label culture bottles.
11. Dispose of contaminated equipment and sharps in appropriate containers.
12. Remove gloves, sanitize hands, and transport specimen to the laboratory.

RELATIONSHIP BETWEEN PROPER LABELING OF BLOOD TUBES AND SENTINEL EVENTS

Sentinel events are those that involve death, permanent impairment, or severe temporary impairment. A blood-related sentinel event is a hemolytic transfusion reaction associated with blood incompatibility, which is most commonly is caused by a failure to properly identify the patient or the blood product. For this reason, labeling of blood bank specimens, usually collected in pink-capped EDTA tubes, should include:

- Patient's full name, including middle name
- Patient's ID number
- Patient's birthdate
- Date and time of sample collection
- Initials of phlebotomist
- Room and bed number (optional)

Two identifiers should always be used to verify the correct patient. Blood bank armbands, with or without barcoding, may be issued to patients when blood is typed and cross-matched, and the number on the armband must be visible.

HANDLING AND PRESERVING EXTRAVASCULAR BODY FLUIDS FOR CHEMICAL ANALYSIS

Amniotic fluid	Store in special container (protected from light) at room temperature for chromosome analysis or on ice for some chemistry tests (according to protocol).
Cerebrospinal fluid	Collect in 3 tubes and store at room temperature with immediate delivery to lab.
Gastric fluids	Store in sterile container at room temperature for up to 6 hours, refrigerated for up to 7 days and frozen for up to 30 days.
Nasopharyngeal secretions.	Place swab in tube with transport medium.
Saliva	Test immediately (point of care) or freeze for hormone tests to maintain stability.
Semen	Keep warm and deliver immediately for testing.
Serous fluids	Place in sterile container for C&S, EDTA tube for cell counts/smears, oxalate or fluoride tubes for chemistry tests.
Synovial fluid	Place in ETDA or heparin tube for cell counts, smear, and crystal identification; sterile tube for C&S; and plain tube for chemistry and immunology tests.
Urine	Store at room temperature in sterile container for 2 hours (protected from light) and then refrigerate. If both UA and C&S required, then test or refrigerate immediately.

GLUCOSE TOLERANCE TEST PROCEDURE

The **glucose tolerance test** (GTT) is used to diagnose disorders of carbohydrate (specifically glucose) metabolism and the ability to metabolize glucose. Procedure:

- Verify patient identification with 2 identifiers.
- Advise patient to drink only water during the procedure and no other beverages, food, or chewing gum, and to avoid smoking.
- Use standard precautions and venipuncture procedures.
- Carry out blood draw (fasting) and check glucose results. Tests is usually not done if fasting glucose is >200 mg/dL.
- Collect a fasting urine specimen if ordered.
- Administer glucose (usually in beverage form over 5 minutes), typically 75 g for adults, 1 g/kg for children or exceptionally small adults, and 50-75 g for pregnant women.
- Start timing and give patient schedule for collections, usually at 30 minutes, 60 minutes, 2 hours and/or 3 hours, depending on the version of the GTT ordered (usually 1-hour, 2-hour, or 3-hour).
- Collect blood and urine (if ordered) specimens according to schedule.
- Label specimens and transport to laboratory.

PROCESSING IRRETRIEVABLE SPECIMENS

Irretrievable specimens are those that require invasive procedures for collection or those that cannot be collected again and include Pap smears, meconium, placenta, cerebrospinal fluid, ascitic/pleural, peritoneal fluid, synovial fluid, and tissue samples, autopsy samples, bronchial lavage samples, urinary stone samples, bone marrow sample, pre-dialysis and pre-drug level samples, and specimens from tissue banks and eye banks. Irretrievable specimens should be labeled with at least 2 identifiers and handled carefully to avoid preanalytical, analytical, and postanalytical errors, and any waste of the sample. Protocols for each type of specimen should be followed exactly, including the time to processing, the method of transport, preservation methods, and processing procedures. For example, CSF should never be refrigerated and should be processed within 30 to 60 minutes of collection to avoid degradation of sample. Irretrievable specimens should be placed in specially labeled specimen bags for transport to the laboratory to alert personnel. The bag should be labeled with the necessary transport/storage temperature (room, iced, frozen, refrigerated).

WAIVED TESTING IN THE CLINICAL LABORATORY

While laboratory testing is regulated by CLIA and results monitored through proficiency testing, some tests are considered to have a very low risk of error (although not necessarily error free), and the patient is unlikely to experience harm if a result is in error. These tests do not require proficiency testing. **Waived testing** includes specific tests exempted by CLIA regulations, tests approved by the FDA for home use (such as pregnancy tests), and tests for which the FDA has applied a waiver based on CLIA regulations and guidelines. Labs that carry out only waived testing must obtain a CLIA Certificate of Waiver (COW). Waived tests include dipstick or tablet reagent tests (such as for bilirubin and ketones), fecal-occult blood tests, blood glucose monitoring strips, ovulation tests (color-based), ESR tests, blood counts, and hemoglobin. Some states may require proficiency testing for tests that are waived under CLIA regulations, and some laboratories may choose to have proficiency testing of waived tests for internal quality control.

Clinical Chemistry

CLINICAL CHEMISTRY TERMINOLOGY

Electrophoresis	Application of electric field to liquid applied to a medium to separate different macromolecules, such as proteins, RNA and DNA, by size and/or charge. Used for analysis of DNA, to determine the presence of proteins and antibody reactions, and to test antibiotics and vaccines.
Chemiluminescence	Light produced by a chemical reaction, such as when applying luminol to blood and observing under darkness. With a chemiluminescence assay, a light-emitting molecule is used to label an antigen or antibody in order to measure the antigen-antibody complex.
Enzyme-linked immunosorbent assay (ELISA)	Plate-based assay utilizes antibodies and color to identify agents (such as antigens or antibodies). Used to determine the presence of antibodies to infections (such as HIV), allergens, hormones (pregnancy testing), or drugs (such as cocaine).
Fluorescence polarization immunoassay (FPIA)	Antibody labeled with fluorescence and combined with a sample believed to contain an antigen and polarized light applied to identify and measure the amount of antigen that binds to the labeled antibody. Used for drug testing and therapeutic drug monitoring.
Spectrophotometry	Measures absorption of light and quantity of coloring matter in a solution to determine composition. May be used to measure activity of enzymes, concentration of protein, bilirubin, glucose, and hemoglobin in serum.
Densitometry	Measures density of liquids and optical density in materials that are light sensitive. Used for DEXA bone scans.
Refractometry	Measures refractive index, how light goes through a substance, to identify composition and purity. Used to identify liquids, components, or characteristics, such as urine specific gravity and serum proteins.
Turbidimetry	Determines the concentration of solutions by how much light is absorbed by particles, which is dependent on the size and number of particles. Used to determine total protein, amylase activity, and lipase activity.
Nephelometry	Measures scattered light in a solution. Used to determine concentration of liquids with antigen-antibody reactions for a variety of lab tests, including immunoglobulins, serum proteins, hemoglobin, albumin, and C-reactive protein.
Osmometry	Measures osmolality of solution, compound, or colloid, such as serum or urine.

35

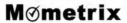

Chromatography	Uses a solid, gas, or liquid to separate a mixture into components in a 2-phase system (stationary and mobile) in which different components go through the medium at different speeds. Gas chromatography is used to detect drugs and alcohol in blood.
Mass spectrometry	Measures the masses found in a sample by converting molecules to ions and separating them and measuring and displaying them graphically. Used to analyze respiratory gases, genomic studies, and newborn screening.

PHOSPHORESCENCE

Phosphorescence: A type of photoluminescence in which radiation from an energy source that is absorbed and stored by particular substance is discharged slowly, and on a continuous basis as light. The radiation is not discharged immediately upon absorption. The light released is the result of an excited electron dropping back down to a lower energy state.

FLUORESCENCE

Fluorescence: A type of photoluminescence in which light is released instantaneously from the movement of an electron from an excited energy state back down to a lower energy state. An energy source, such as ultraviolet light, is what "excites" an electron of an atom initially. In fluorescence, the light released has a longer wavelength than the light that was initially absorbed.

BIOLUMINESCENCE

Bioluminescence: A type of luminescence in which a chemical reaction is responsible for the excitation energy needed to raise an electron from its lower energy state to a higher energy state. When the excited electron falls back to a lower energy state, an emission of light is produced. The particular chemical reaction related to bioluminescence is one in which oxygen reacts with luciferin. The enzyme luciferase must be present for the resulting bioluminescence.

CLINICAL LABORATORY INSTRUMENTATION TERMINOLOGY

Radiant energy	Electromagnetic and gravitational energy that travels by waves or particles, such as heat from the sun or other sources, x-rays, and gamma rays. Commonly used for diagnostic (radiographs) and therapeutic purposes (radiation therapy).
End-point reactions	Completion of a chemical reaction. For example, the end-point reaction for a reagent strip is when it changes color.
Diffraction grating	Splitting of a ray of white light into component colors. Used in DIC microscopy and with monochromators to analyze biopsy specimens.
Kinetic/rate reactions	Used to measure the rate of change or concentration associated with creation of a product or loss of a substrate. Measures analytes, such as enzymes and ammonia, and is used for enzyme tests such as lipase and alanine aminotransferase.
Random access	Ability to access data in random order rather than sequential.

PHOTOMULTIPLIER TUBE

A photomultiplier tube converts light to electrical currents. This conversion to electricity is extremely rapid. In addition, the tube amplifies the signal that is received. This amplification can be

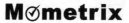

very high, up to one million times amplification. To accomplish this conversion, as well as the amplification, a very high internal voltage must be present. The voltage can be as high as 1500 volts.

TURBIDIMETRY AND ITS INHERENT PROBLEMS

Turbidimetry is a measurement of the quantity of light that is blocked by particles in a solution as the light passes through that solution (turbidity). There are several problems inherent in this technique, however. In order to compare the turbidity of a sample with a standard, the quantity and number of particles present in both the sample and the standard must be similar or comparable. Any great variation in particle size between the particles present in the sample and the particles present in the standard can be problematic. Also, any settling and/or aggregation of particles present can be a problem in obtaining accurate results. Consistent timing in the preparation of the samples is therefore extremely necessary to avoid this issue.

FLAME EMISSION PHOTOMETRY

Flame emission photometry is based on the fact that excited electrons release extra energy (light) when the electrons drop down to their stable ground state. For example, when a metallic element (such as Na+, K+, or Li+) absorbs energy (in the form of heat), the orbital electrons of that element move to a higher, unstable energy level from the stable ground state. These electrons are now called "excited electrons". Since the excited electrons are at an unstable energy level, the drop back down to their ground state, to achieve a stable energy. As the electrons do this, they release their extra energy in the form of light. The light is released at a specific wavelength, depending on the element in question. Each element has a unique wavelength associated with it. Furthermore, the quantity of light that is released is directly related to the amount of the particular element present.

VARIOUS STATIONARY AND MOVING PHASES

HIGH PERFORMANCE LIQUID CHROMATOGRAPHY (HPLC)

Stationary phase: liquid adsorbed on the column packing

Moving phase: liquid pumped through the column

THIN LAYER CHROMATOGRAPHY (TLC)

Stationary phase: a thin layer of silica gel that is spread on a piece of plastic or glass

Moving phase: a solvent that uses capillary action to move along a piece of paper

GAS-LIQUID CHROMATOGRAPHY (GLC)

Stationary phase: liquid adsorbed on particles packed in a column

Moving phase: a gas that travels through the column

PAPER CHROMATOGRAPHY

Stationary phase: the paper where the sample is placed

Moving phase: a solvent that uses capillary action to move along a piece of paper

MASS SPECTROMETRY

Mass spectrometry is a technique used in the identification of compounds. This identification is accomplished using a mass spectrometer. A mass spectrometer determines the mass (molecular weight) to charge ratio of ions in the sample being tested. A mass spectrum can then be created which shows the masses of the components (ions) present in the sample. In the creation of the mass spectrum, magnetic and/or electric fields are used to sort the ions. Mass spectrometry is useful in identifying drugs in the lab, and it can be used in conjunction with a variety of other laboratory techniques, such as gas-liquid chromatography.

USING MASS SPECTROMETRY IN CONJUNCTION WITH GAS-LIQUID CHROMATOGRAPHY

Mass spectrometry can be used in conjunction with gas-liquid chromatography in the lab to aid the technician in the proper identification of a sample. Certain compounds, albeit different compounds from each other, can have similar retention times. Gas-liquid chromatography uses retention times to identify compounds. Therefore, if several compounds have similar retention times, the compound in question can be misidentified using gas-liquid chromatography alone. However, if the peak resulting from a gas-liquid chromatography analysis is taken to a mass spectrometer for analysis on the basis of mass, the particular compound in question can be correctly identified.

ELECTROLYTIC CELL

An electrolytic cell consists of three main parts: an anode, a cathode, and an electrolytic solution. When electricity is applied to an electrolytic cell, an internal chemical reaction in the cell between the ions present in the electrolytic solution and the anode or cathode occurs. The electrolytic solution is composed of water and other solvents, for the purpose of dissolving ions in the solution. The anode is a positively charged electrode, and negatively charged ions (anions) flow toward the anode. These ions are oxidized, or lose electrons, at the anode. The cathode is a negatively charged electrode, and positively charged ions (cations) flow toward the cathode. These ions are reduced, or gain electrons, at the cathode.

OSMOMETER OPERATION

Osmometers measure the osmotic pressure, vapor pressure, and osmotic strength of solutions. Many different types of osmometers (vapor pressure depression, freezing point depression, membrane) are available and may operate slightly differently. Osmometers are commonly used to assess the concentrations (osmolality) of salts and sugars present in blood of urine:

1. Gather reagents and equipment.
2. Follow manufacturers guidelines for calibration (often done automatically) with sampler, which usually requires analysis of 2 calibration standards. Calibration standards include 1500 mOsm/kg and 850 mOsm/kg. Complete calibration and utilize chamber cleaner if needed.
3. Draw sample into sampler and insert sampler into testing chamber.
4. Press start button and wait for results, remove sampler and clean chamber.

NEPHELOMETER OPERATION

Nephelometers measure concentration of particulates in gas or liquid. In medicine, nephelometry is used to measure the levels of blood protein (immunoglobulins) when assessing immune function and can detect antigens or antibodies with a light beam (usually laser) according to light-scattering properties. Nephelometers are commonly used outside of medicine to measure air quality, including visibility. Many different types of nephelometers are available and may operate slightly differently:

1. Gather supplies.
2. Calibrate with standard at 1:80, 1:160 and continue doubling to 1:2560 according to manufacturer's guidelines
3. Load specimen into serum racks and reagent into reagent racks.
4. Adjust equipment to proper setting for test.

5. Run sample.
6. Remove sample and reagent.
7. Shut down equipment.

IMMUNOASSAY AND ELECTROPHORESIS PRINCIPLES

Immunoassays utilize antigens or antibodies to test for the presence of disease. For example, an antigen may be used to test for the presence of antibodies in a blood sample. If present, the antibody will bind to the antigen. Immunoassays that identify target antibodies include tests for rheumatoid factor, West Nile virus, and hepatitis B. Immunoassays that target antigens include tests for levels of drugs (digoxin), levels of hormones (testosterone, insulin), and markers of cancer (PSA).

Electrophoresis involves application of an electrical field to macromolecules (RNA, DNA, and proteins) suspended in liquid on various media in order to separate them by size. A charge (negative or positive) causes macromolecules to move toward the opposite charge. Electrophoresis may be used to study DNA or RNA and may help to diagnosis disorders that involve abnormal proteins, such as some types of cancer, renal disease, and multiple sclerosis. Electrophoresis is also used to test vaccines and antibiotics.

PERFORMING PREVENTIVE MAINTENANCE ON LABORATORY EQUIPMENT

A medical technologist should perform preventive maintenance for several reasons. For one, as equipment is used, parts can tend to wear out or even break. For best equipment performance, these worn out parts should be replaced regularly. Calibration and other adjustments should also be made on a regular basis so equipment can give the most accurate results in laboratory tests. Preventive maintenance is also important for keeping instruments and equipment clean. Following all preventive maintenance schedules will keep laboratory equipment running smoothly, and will also keep all equipment functioning for as long as possible.

DISCRETE ANALYZERS VS. CONTINUOUS FLOW ANALYZERS

A discrete analyzer is an analyzer in which all specimens and samples are analyzed separately. The specimens each have their own individual vessels for analysis. An example of a discrete analyzer is the Automated Clinical Analyzer (ACA). A continuous flow analyzer is an analyzer in which all samples flow through the same tubing during analysis. In addition, the samples flow in a continuous stream. To separate the samples analyzed in a continuous flow analyzer, air bubbles are used. An example of a continuous flow analyzer is the Sequential Multiple Analyzer Computer (SMAC).

CHEMISTRY ANALYZER MAINTENANCE

Maintenance of the chemistry analyzer will vary depending on the types and size, with some requiring much more hands-on maintenance and manual calibration than others. General maintenance requirements include:

- Check location of installation (electrical, infrastructure), including voltage, outlet polarity, and space for ventilation and cables.
- Assess security and cleanliness.
- Assess exposure to thermal radiation, vibration, excess humidity, excess temperature, dust, smoke, and corrosive materials/emissions.
- Check any lights and on/off or command buttons to make sure they are functioning.
- Check printer.
- Clean any spills, breakage.
- Ensure equipment is covered when not in use.

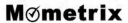
- Ensure proper calibration is carried out.
- If the equipment has fuses, replace as needed.
- For small equipment, ensure it is disconnected from power after use.
- Carry out routine scheduled maintenance, daily, weekly, monthly, every 6 months, and annually according to manufacturer's guidelines.

ACCURACY, RANDOM ERROR, PRECISION, STANDARD DEVIATION, AND VARIANCE

Accuracy: Accuracy refers to the ability of a test to obtain a true (or accurate) value.

Random Error: Random errors are any departures from the true or accurate value. Random errors are caused by errors that are inherent in all laboratory analyses and tests. The causes of random errors are often not able to be determined, and they are often unavoidable.

Precision: Precision is the reproducibility of results obtained from a particular test. If repeated testing provides the same results time after time, then there is said to be a high degree of precision.

Standard Deviation: The standard deviation is a value that estimates the random errors that are inherent in any test or analytical procedure. It gives insight into how much the obtained data values deviate from the mean (or average) data value.

Variance: The variance is the value of standard deviation multiplied by itself (square of the standard deviation). Similar to the standard deviation, it measures how obtained data values are spread around the mean (or average) value.

MODE, MEDIAN, GEOMETRIC MEAN, AND ARITHMETIC MEAN

Mode: The mode is the particular numerical value that is the most frequent in a particular set of numbers.

Median: If a group of numbers are arranged from lowest to highest, according to magnitude, the median is the middle value of the set of numbers.

Geometric Mean: The geometric mean of a group of numbers is calculated by adding all of the logarithms of the numbers in the set of numbers divided by the quantity of numbers in the set. Then, the antilogarithm of this value is taken to obtain the geometric mean.

Arithmetic Mean: The arithmetic mean is usually called the average value. If you add up all of the numbers in a particular group of numbers, and then divide that result by the quantity of numbers in the group, the arithmetic mean is calculated.

QUALITY CONTROL CHART

SHIFTS AND TRENDS

A shift is said to have occurred when the control values on a quality control chart appear to have changed suddenly. Also, if the control values on the quality control chart are consistently being found to be higher or lower than the mean value (within two standard deviations) on several days in a row in the laboratory, a shift is said to have occurred. A trend on a quality control chart, on the other hand, is a gradual, fairly slow change in control values over a time period of several days. This is in contrast to the abrupt change in control values that characterizes a shift.

CAUSES OF UPWARD SHIFTS, DOWNWARD SHIFTS, TRENDS

An upward shift on a quality control chart may be caused by the change to a new standard that has a lower concentration than what is required for the particular test being performed. A downward shift, on the other hand, can be caused by the change to a new standard that has a higher concentration than what is required for the particular test being performed. A trend on a quality control chart is most often caused by a slow deterioration or breaking down of an instrument, piece of equipment, or a reagent. A trend can be either downwards or upwards.

QUALITY ASSURANCE

Quality assurance involves the monitoring and checking of all aspects of the medical laboratory. A laboratory quality assurance program involves several aspects. For one, all instruments and equipment should be checked on a regular basis. Making sure that all parts are in working order and are performing as expected is very important. This is also a part of the preventive maintenance program. Specimen collection and labeling should also be monitored. Correct collection and labeling of specimens is an important step in obtaining accurate laboratory results. All laboratory supplies, equipment, and even water should also be reviewed. All supplies should meet all necessary specifications, and should be in found in working order. Finally, the precision and accuracy of all laboratory results and analyses should be a priority. Quality control charts, appropriate controls and standards should all be used. A laboratory's participation in an external survey program, such as one from the American Society of Clinical Pathologists (ASCP) will also help a laboratory maintain its quality assurance.

STANDARD AND CONTROL

Standard: A material, such as a serum, that has a known composition, and a high degree of purity. Standards are used to identify and describe other materials or samples. A standard is often described by its chemical and physical character. Laboratory standards are often available from the National Bureau of Standards.

Control: A control is a substance that contains known concentrations and amounts of the materials that will be measured in a particular test. The control will often have a chemical and physical character that is similar to sample being tested.

PROCEDURES FOR HANDLING OUT OF CONTROL TEST RESULTS

When a group of test results appears to be out of control, the troubleshooting procedures for the test method in question must be followed. As part of the laboratory's quality control program, these troubleshooting procedures should already be written and developed for use in cases such as these. The instructions will likely tell the technician to check any and all calculations that have been made, to make a visual inspection of all reagents that have been used, and to inspect all instruments and equipment that have been used as well. After these steps have been accomplished to satisfaction, the technician may be instructed to rerun a set of tests with a new sample of the control. In discovering a group of out of control test results, the technician is not to inform the doctor ordering the tests of the out of control results. Also, the technician should be sure to not change batches of standards or reagents used, as this will affect the results obtained.

FORMATION OF CREATININE

Creatinine is formed from free creatine. Creatine is formed from various amino acids, including glycine, arginine, and methionine. Guanidoacetate is formed from a reaction between glycine and arginine in various body tissues, including the liver, pancreas, and the kidneys. The guanidoacetate is moved to the liver via the blood, where it reacts with S-adenosylmethionine to form creatine. The creatine is then transported to various muscle tissues via the blood system. This creatine is found in the form of phosphocreatine in the muscle tissues. Phosphocreatine is a high energy compound and helps form ATP by supplying phosphate for the formation. ATP is very important for muscle metabolism. When the ATP is formed, there is also a release of free creatine. The free creatine then

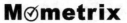

transforms in the creatinine through an irreversible and spontaneous reaction. Creatinine is excreted as a waste product in human urine, and serves no functional purpose in the human body.

RENAL FUNCTION TESTS

Non-protein nitrogens: Creatinine, BUN, uric acid, and ammonia	Collect 1 mL serum in red or tiger-capped tube or 1 mL plasma in heparinized green-capped tube. <u>Uric acid</u>—If patient is receiving rasburicase, the specimen must be obtained in a pre-chilled heparinized tube and transported in ice slurry. <u>Ammonia</u>—1 mL plasma in EDTA lavender capped tube or heparinized green-capped tube (tightly capped) and transported in ice slurry. Method of testing for all: Spectrophotometry.
Creatinine clearance Reference value: 70-130 mL/min/1.73^2	Patients should avoid strenuous exercise for 48 hours before beginning test and meat/other protein restricted to ≤8 ounces for 24 hours before beginning test. Collection begins after disposing of first morning urine. A blood specimen is usually also taken for a serum creatinine. Urine is collected for a 24-hour period and stored at room temperature. Urine is mixed and measured and a specimen transferred for creatinine testing. Data are entered into computer (age, height, weight, ethnicity if appropriate).
Estimated glomerular filtration rate (eGFR) Reference value: >90 mL/min/1.73^2 <60 ml/min/1.73^2 indicates kidney disease	The eGFR is not directly measured but is estimated based on serum creatinine levels. Various formulas are used to estimate the GFR: General (adults): (Urine Creatinine / Serum Creatinine) × Urine Volume (mL) / [time (hr) X 60] = eGFR. Schwartz (children): (k) × height in cm/ serum creatinine = GFR (mL/min/1.73m^2). k = Constant (muscle mass) k = 0.33 in premature infants k = 0.45 in term infants to 1 year old k = 0.55 in children to 13 years and adolescent females k = 0.65 in adolescent males <u>Modified MDRD formula for 18-70 years</u>: GFR (mL/min/1.73 m^2) = 175 x (Scr)$^{-1.154}$ x (Age)$^{-0.203}$ x (0.742 if female) x (1.212 if African American) (conventional units).

RENAL FUNCTION TESTS AND CORRELATION WITH PATHOLOGICAL CONDITIONS AFFECTING KIDNEY FUNCTION

Specific gravity	1.015-1.025. Determines kidney's ability to concentrate urinary solutes. <u>Increased</u>: dehydration, diabetes, fever, CHF, and adrenal insufficiency. <u>Decreased</u>: diuresis, hypervolemia, hypothermia, and renal disease (impaired concentrating ability)
Osmolality (urine)	350-900 mOsm/kg/24 hours. Shows early defects if kidney's ability to concentrate urine is impaired. <u>Increased</u>: CHF, dehydration, SIADH, and azotemia. <u>Decreased</u>: diabetes insipidus, hypernatremia, hypokalemia, and primary polydipsia.
Osmolality (serum)	275-295 mOsm/kg. <u>Increased</u>: Azotemia, dehydration, diabetes insipidus, diabetic ketoacidosis, hypercalcemia, and hypernatremia. <u>Decreased</u>: adrenocorticoid insufficiency, hyponatremia, SIADH, and water intoxication.

Creatinine clearance (24-hour)	Male 85-125 mL/min/1.73 m², Female 75-115 mL/min/1.73 m². Evaluates the amount of blood cleared of creatinine in 1 minute. Approximates the glomerular filtration rate.
Serum creatinine	0.6-1.2 mg/dL. Level should remain stable with normal functioning. Increased: acromegaly, CHF, poliomyelitis, renal disease, shock, and rhabdomyolysis. Decreased: loss of muscle mass, hyperthyroidism, inadequate protein intake, liver disease, muscular dystrophy, and pregnancy.
Urine creatinine	Male 14-26 mg/kg/24 hr, Female 11-20 mg/kg/24 hr. Increased: acromegaly, carnivorous diets, exercise, and gigantism. Decreased: glomerulonephritis, pyelonephritis, leukemia, muscle wasting disorders, PKD, shock, urinary tract obstructions, and vegetarian diets.
Blood urea nitrogen (BUN)	7-8 mg/dL (8-20 mg/dL >60 years of age). Increased: impaired renal function (as urea is end product of protein metabolism), chronic glomerulonephritis, CHF, diabetes, GI bleeding, hypovolemia, ketoacidosis, starvation (muscle wasting), neoplasm, pyelonephritis, shock, nephrotoxic agents, and urinary tract obstruction. Decreased: inadequate protein intake, low protein diet, malabsorption syndromes, pregnancy, and liver disease.
BUN/creatinine ratio	10:1. Increases with hypovolemia. With intrinsic kidney disease, the ratio is normal, but the BUN and creatinine are increased.
Uric acid	Male 4.4-7.6, Female 2.3-6.6 mg/dL. Increased: renal failure, gout, pernicious anemia, and sickle cell anemia. Decreased: chronic alcoholism, hypertension, and renal disease.

JAFFE REACTION FOR CREATININE DETERMINATION

The Jaffe reaction is the basis for most creatinine determination methods. It is based on the fact that creatinine reacts with an alkaline picrate solution. This reaction produces a bright orange-red compound, indicating the presence of creatinine. There is a major drawback to the Jaffe reaction, however. This drawback is that it has a lack of specificity for creatinine. Several other compounds can react with an alkaline picrate solution, such as glucose and various proteins. Using Lloyd's reagent can help with this drawback however. Lloyd's reagent is an aluminum silicate that can adsorb creatinine. This aids in the separation of creatinine from some of the competing compounds before the development of the orange-red compound.

MATHEMATICAL EQUATION FOR CREATININE CLEARANCE FOR AN AVERAGE SIZED ADULT

The creatinine clearance for an average sized adult, in milliliters per minute (mL/min), can be calculated by the equation U/P x V. In this equation, U represents the creatinine concentration in the urine, in milligrams per deciliter (mg/dL), P represents the creatinine concentration in the plasma, in milligrams per deciliter (mg/dL), and V represents the volume of urine per minute, with the volume expressed in milliliters. Use the conversion factor of 24 hours being equal to 1440 minutes to convert the volume of urine over a 24 hour period to the volume of urine per minute. One thing to keep in mind with calculating the creatinine clearance is that the body surface area and the kidney size of an individual can affect the creatinine clearance. In an average sized individual, these factors are not really taken into account.

ALTERING THE MATHEMATICAL EQUATION FOR CALCULATING CREATININE CLEARANCE FOR AN INFANT

When calculating creatinine clearance for an infant, we need to take into account the body surface area of the infant. Therefore, use the equation U/P x V x 1.73/A to calculate the creatinine clearance of an infant (mL/min/standard surface area). In this equation, U represents the creatinine concentration in the urine in milligrams per deciliter (mg/dL), P represents the creatinine concentration in the plasma in milligrams per deciliter (mg/dL), and V represents the volume of urine per minute with the volume expressed in milliliters. Use the conversion factor of 24 hours being equal to 1440 minutes to convert the volume of urine over a 24 hour period to the volume of urine per minute. 1.73 represents the average body surface area in square meters (m^2) of an average sized adult. A is the body surface area in square meters (m^2) of the individual (the infant) in question.

ULTRAVIOLET PROCEDURE FOR QUANTIFYING URIC ACID

The ultraviolet procedure for quantifying uric acid is based on the principle that uric acid absorbs ultraviolet light in the region of 290—293 nm. If uricase is added to uric acid, the uricase will destroy the uric acid. This happens because the uricase acts as a catalyst helping to break down the uric acid to carbon dioxide and allantoin. Because of this breakdown and the ability of uric acid to absorb ultraviolet light, differential spectrophotometry can be used to quantify uric acid in a sample. The ultraviolet procedure is accomplished using centrifugal fast-analyzer systems. These systems have the ability to monitor the decreasing absorbance of ultraviolet light as the uric acid is destroyed by uricase. As the uric acid is destroyed, and its concentration in a specimen decreases, the absorbance of ultraviolet light also proportionally decreases.

ORTHOSTATIC PROTEINURIA

Orthostatic proteinuria (also referred to as postural proteinuria) is a condition that is characterized by an excessive amount of protein (usually albumin) that is excreted into urine as a function of the patient's position. Usually, during the day, when the patient is upright (sitting or standing), there is an increased amount of protein excreted into the urine. At night, however, when the patient is lying down, there is a normal amount of protein excreted into the urine. This condition affects adolescents mostly between the ages of ten and twenty, and up to three to five percent of adolescents are affected with orthostatic proteinuria. Affected people, other than the excessive protein excretion, have no other health problems or issues, and for the most part, appear to be healthy. In the laboratory, the existence of this condition can be determined by comparing urine samples taken during the day, and ones taken at night, or right after a person awakes from sleeping.

ANATOMY AND PHYSIOLOGY OF THE LIVER

The **liver** is a cone-shaped organ in the right upper quadrant of the abdominal cavity, superior to the stomach and inferior to the diaphragm. The liver is encased in a capsule and divided into 2 primary lobes (larger right and smaller left) and 2 minor lobes (quadrate and caudate). The primary lobes contain 8 segments of 1000 lobules, the functional unit. The lobules contain a central vein with hepatic cells radiating outward with sinusoids (vascular channels) separating groups of hepatic cells. In the sinusoids, arterial blood from the hepatic artery mixes with venous blood from the hepatic portal vein, which brings nutrients from the digestive tract. Kupffer cells in the sinusoids remove pathogens from the blood through phagocytosis. The liver produces bile, proteins, and cholesterol, and converts excess glucose into glycogen to store. The liver filters the blood of toxins (including drugs) and bilirubin, regulates blood clotting and levels of amino acids, and produces immune factors to help resist infection. The liver forms urea from ammonia so it can be excreted in the urine.

BILIRUBIN

Bilirubin is the breakdown product that is derived from the degradation of the heme in hemoglobin. It is the reddish-yellow pigment of bile, and it can either be described as being conjugated (water-soluble in blood) or unconjugated (bound to albumin). The formation of bilirubin starts with the breakdown of hemoglobin in old (dying) red blood cells. This breakdown is very rapid in certain cells of the bone marrow, spleen, and liver. First, the globin protein is denatured and removed from the hemoglobin in the red blood cells. Then, the tetrapyrrole ring (4 pyrroles in a ring) of the heme is oxidized and opened up. Iron is then added and the green pigment biliverdin is formed. Biliverdin is then reduced by the addition of hydrogen to form bilirubin.

HEMOGLOBIN

Hemoglobin is an iron-containing protein that is used to transport oxygen from the lungs to other body tissues. The iron in the hemoglobin is what gives blood its characteristic red color. Hemoglobin contains 4 iron atoms, 4 heme groups, and 4 globin chains (or protein groups). Hemoglobin contains approximately 94% globin and 6% heme. In addition, hemoglobin is produced in the bone marrow by erythrocytes. The most common form of hemoglobin in an adult is hemoglobin A.

JAUNDICE

Jaundice is a condition that is characterized by the yellowing of certain parts of the body, such as the skin, the sclera (whites of the eyes) and the mucous membranes. Jaundice is due to an increased amount of bilirubin in the blood plasma. The bilirubin can either be conjugated bilirubin or unconjugated bilirubin (conjugated jaundice or unconjugated jaundice). Jaundice is said to be present when the total bilirubin levels are greater than 2.5 mg/dL. The increased amount of bilirubin in the blood can be due to several things. For one, there could be an obstruction in the bile duct of the liver (obstructive jaundice). There could also be an increase in the breakdown of blood in the body, causing increased bilirubin levels (hemolytic jaundice), or liver cells could be damaged (parenchymal jaundice). Jaundice can also be due to a combination of these factors.

> **Review Video: Jaundice/Icterus**
> Visit mometrix.com/academy and enter code: 339680

HEPATIC FUNCTION TESTS

Procedures	
Bilirubin	Collect sample in heparinized green-capped tube, 0.6 mL blood, centrifuge to volume of 0.2 mL plasma/serum. Sample must be protected from light and analyzed within 2 hours. Refrigerate for storage. Test in chemical analyzer or photometric assay according to manufacturer's directions.
Albumin	Collect sample in red top with or without clot activator or heparinized green-top tube for test on serum or plasma. Test in chemical analyzer according to manufacturer's directions.
Prothrombin time (PT)	Sample should completely fill blue-capped tube with inversions immediately after drawing. Do not centrifuge or freeze if sample must be transported. Test in coagulometer.
Alkaline phosphatase (ALP)	Patient should fast 8-12 hours before test. Sample collected in gel-barrier tube and centrifuged as soon as possible for complete separation. Test in chemical analyzer.

Procedures	
Aspartate aminotransferase (AST)	Sample collected in gel-barrier tube, centrifuged for complete separation, and stored in refrigerator. Test in chemical analyzer according to manufacturer's directions.
Alanine transferase (ALT)	Same as AST.
Gamma-glutamyl transpeptidase (GGT)	Same as AST. Separate as soon as possible.
Ammonia	Sample collected in 1 mL plasma in EDTA lavender capped tube or heparinized green-capped tube (tightly capped) and transported in ice slurry. Centrifuge within 15 minutes without removing stopper, separate plasma and freeze in plastic vial. Test through micro-diffusion apparatus (indirect), enzymatic method (direct) with glutamate dehydrogenase or ammonium electrode, or ammonia analyzer.
Cholesterol	Patient should fast for 12 hours. Collect sample in red top with or without clot activator or heparinized green-top tube for test on serum or plasma. Store serum in refrigerator. Test in analyzer.

HEPATIC FUNCTION TESTS AND CORRELATION WITH PATHOLOGICAL CONDITIONS

Results	
Bilirubin	Determines the ability of the liver to conjugate and excrete bilirubin: direct 0.0-0.3 mg/dL, total 0.0-0.9 mg/dL, and urine 0. Increased: Hemolytic jaundice, hemolytic anemia, liver disease, anorexia nervosa, hypothyroidism, and obstructive jaundice.
Albumin	Albumin: 4.0-5.5 g/dL. Primary protein found in the liver. Decreased: Liver disease, malabsorption, malnutrition, chronic diseases, parasitic infections, prolonged immobilization, burns, kidney disease, pre-eclampsia, overhydration, Cushing disease, and enteropathies. Albumin/globulin (A/G) ratio: 1.5:1 to 2.5:1. Albumin should be greater than globulin. Abnormalities occur with liver disease.
Prothrombin time (PT)	100% or clot detection in 10 to 13 seconds. Increased: Liver disease, coagulation disorders, massive transfusions, celiac disease, salicylate overdose, vitamin K deficiency, and chronic diarrhea. Decreased: Ovarian hyperfunction and ileitis.
Alkaline phosphatase (ALP)	17-142 adults. (Normal values vary with method.) Indicates biliary tract obstruction if no bone disease. Increased: Liver tumor, hepatitis, aplastic anemia, Hodgkin disease, multiple myeloma, polycythemia vera, leukemias, thrombocytopenia. Decreased: Sickle cell and sideroblastic anemia.
Aspartate aminotransferase (AST)	10-40 units. Increased: Liver cell damage, hepatitis, pancreatitis, shock, cardiac arrhythmias, CHF, muscle disease, MI, CVA, and DTs. Decreased: Hemodialysis, vitamin B-6 deficiency, and uremia.
Alanine transferase (ALT)	5-35 units. Increased: Liver cell damage, pancreatitis, AIDS, burns, muscle injury, muscular dystrophy, myositis, shock, and pre-eclampsia. Decreased: Pyridoxal phosphate deficiency.
Gamma-glutamyl transpeptidase (GGT)	5-55 µ/L females, 5-85 µ/L males. Increased: Alcohol abuse, liver disease, hyperthyroidism, mononucleosis, pancreatitis, and renal transplantation. Decreased: Hypothyroidism.

Results	
Lactate dehydrogenase (LDH)	100-200 units. Increased: Alcohol abuse, hepatic carcinoma, hemolytic anemias, leukemias, MI or pulmonary infarction, pancreatitis, shock, viral hepatitis, and renal disease.
Serum ammonia	150-250 mg/dL. Increased: Liver failure, GI hemorrhage, inborn deficiency, and total parenteral nutrition.
Cholesterol	<200 mg/dL. Increased: Bile duct obstruction, diabetes, glomerulonephritis, gout, hypothyroidism, nephrotic syndrome, obesity, pregnancy, syndrome X, and anorexia nervosa. Decreased: Hepatic parenchymal disease, pernicious anemia, hyperthyroidism, COPD, leukemia (CML), thalassemia, sideroblastic anemia, and myeloma.

ELEVATED TEST VALUES IN LIVER DISEASE, OBSTRUCTIVE JAUNDICE, AND HEMOLYTIC JAUNDICE

Cirrhosis	Generally, values of hepatic function tests elevated. Creatinine clearance falls with hepatorenal syndrome and serum creatinine increases; ammonia levels increase with hepatic encephalopathy.
Liver failure	Elevation of AST, GGT, ALT, ASP, lactate, ammonia, and bilirubin.
Viral hepatitis	Elevation of bilirubin (serum and urine), ALP may elevate with biliary obstruction/abscess, PT may be prolonged. Serum ammonia may be elevated (with altered mental status). AST, ALT, and GTT may be elevated.
Obstructive jaundice	Serum bilirubin, ALP, and GTT are elevated. AST is usually not elevated unless complications occur. PT may be prolonged. Urine bilirubin is usually not present.
Hemolytic jaundice	Elevation of unconjugated bilirubin and LDH.

DETERMINING SERUM BILIRUBIN CONCENTRATION

Bilirubin Oxidase: In this method, bilirubin oxidase, an enzyme, serves as a catalyst in the oxidation of bilirubin to biliverdin. This oxidation is characterized by a decrease in absorbance from 405—460 nm.

Bilirubinometer: In this method, a bilirubinometer is used to read bilirubin concentration at 454 nm. The bilirubinometer is used as a direct spectrophotometric assay.

Jendrassik-Grof: In this method, the coupling reaction of unconjugated bilirubin with the diazo reagent is accelerated with a caffeine-sodium benzoate mixture. This coupling reaction forms an azobilirubin complex, which can be used to determine bilirubin concentration in the sample. This method is the preferred method to use when determining serum bilirubin concentration, for it has a high recovery rate.

Malloy-Evelyn: This particular method uses alcohol to dissolve unconjugated bilirubin. The unconjugated bilirubin then reacts with diazotized sulfanilic acid.

GILBERT'S SYNDROME

Gilbert's Syndrome is an inherited disorder that is characterized by the presence of an abnormal liver enzyme. This particular enzyme is necessary for the disposal of bilirubin. People with this syndrome have a problem with their hepatic uptake of bilirubin because this liver enzyme is abnormal. This syndrome is characterized by an increased level of unconjugated bilirubin, and a

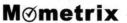

slightly elevated level of bilirubin in the blood. Mild jaundice is a side effect of this syndrome. The illness is often harmless, so often no treatment is required for people with Gilbert's Syndrome.

DUBIN-JOHNSON SYNDROME

Dubin-Johnson Syndrome: In this syndrome, the transport of conjugated bilirubin is defective, and there is an impairment of the excretion of bilirubin in the bile. This leads to an increased level of conjugated (direct) bilirubin in serum, as well as an increased amount of bilirubin in the urine. There is no accompanying increase in the elevation of liver enzymes.

CRIGLER-NAJJAR SYNDROME

Crigler-Najjar Syndrome: This syndrome is characterized by an enzyme deficiency. The enzyme uridine diphosphate glucuronyl transferase is responsible for conjugating bilirubin. People with this syndrome are, therefore, unable to conjugate bilirubin, and an increased level of unconjugated bilirubin is displayed. Crigler-Najjar Syndrome is a hereditary disorder.

TERMINOLOGY OF CARBOHYDRATE METABOLISM

Carbohydrate	Class of nutrients comprised of carbon, hydrogen, and oxygen, and include simple carbohydrates (1 or 2 sugar molecules) or complex carbohydrates (multiple sugar molecules). Monosaccharides (1 sugar molecule) include glucose, fructose, and galactose. Disaccharides (2 linked monosaccharides) include sucrose, maltose, and lactose. Polysaccharides (thousands of linked glucose molecules) include starch, glycogen, and fiber, and do not taste sweet.
Ketones	Organic compound produced by the liver from fatty acids.
Lipogenesis	Metabolic process by which simple sugars are converted to fatty acids or triglycerides for storage.
Renal threshold (glucose)	The glucose level at which the proximal tubule can no longer reabsorb glucose and it spills into the urine for excretion, usually when glucose levels reach 160-180 mg/dL.

POLYSACCHARIDES, DISACCHARIDES, AND MONOSACCHARIDES

Polysaccharide: A polysaccharide is a carbohydrate molecule that is made up of a number of monosaccharide molecules that have been joined together through condensation (the loss of water). The bonds joining the monosaccharides in a polysaccharide are often called glycosidic bonds. An example of a polysaccharide is a starch.

Disaccharide: A carbohydrate (sugar) that is composed of two monosaccharide molecules. Disaccharides are formed by condensation, or the loss of water. An example of a disaccharide is sucrose.

Monosaccharide: A carbohydrate that cannot be broken down further by hydrolysis. Monosaccharides are often called simple sugars. They have a general chemical formula of $C_n (H_2O)_n$. An example of a monosaccharide is glucose.

GLYCOGENESIS, GLYCOGENOLYSIS, GLYCOLYSIS, AND GLUCONEOGENESIS

Glycogenesis: Glycogenesis is the formation of glycogen from blood glucose. The glycogen is formed in the liver, and is due to high glucose levels in the blood.

Glycogenolysis: Glycogenolysis is the hydrolysis (or breaking down) of glycogen to glucose. This reaction takes place in the liver and in muscle tissue. It is due to low blood glucose levels.

Glycolysis: Glycolysis is the metabolism of glucose to pyruvate and lactate (or pyruvic acid). This reaction releases energy.

Gluconeogenesis: Gluconeogenesis is the reaction in which noncarbohydrate sources in the body (such as fat and proteins) form glucose. This reaction takes place in primarily in the liver.

KETONE BODIES

Ketone bodies: Substances containing ketone that are produced through a process called ketogenesis. In ketogenesis, ketone bodies are produced from the breaking down of fatty acids to produce energy. This degradation of fatty acids takes place in the cells of the liver. The ketone bodies are produced from acetyl coenzyme A (CoA) in the liver. Ketogenesis occurs when there are no or very few carbohydrates for the body to use to produce energy. This situation occurs most frequently due to starvation or uncontrolled Type I diabetes. Ketone bodies accumulate in the urine and the blood of such individuals. Examples of ketone bodies are acetone, acetoacetic acid, and beta-hydroxybutyric acid.

HYDROLYSIS

Hydrolysis is a chemical reaction of a molecule with water. Hydrolysis will result in the formation of new molecules. For example, if a molecule of disaccharide is hydrolyzed, the reaction will result in the formation of two monosaccharide molecules. Maltose, lactose, and sucrose are all disaccharides, and their hydrolysis each results in two monosaccharides. The hydrolysis of maltose results in two glucose molecules. The hydrolysis of a molecule of lactose results in the formation of a molecule of galactose and a molecule of glucose. And, finally, the hydrolysis of a molecule of sucrose results in the formation of a molecule of both fructose and a molecule of glucose.

TYPES OF DIABETES

Pre-diabetes	Occurs when blood glucose levels increase above normal (110-126 mg/dL). Patients typically exhibit insulin resistance.
Diabetes mellitus, type 1	Results from destruction of pancreatic beta cells that normally produce insulin. Because insulin is not available, the liver cannot store glucose and hyperglycemia occurs, resulting in osmotic diuresis. The cells cannot utilize glucose for nourishment, and protein and fat break down, leading to ketoacidosis. Insulin is the primary treatment. Most common in children and adults <40.
Diabetes mellitus, type 2	Results from inadequate production of glucose and eventual hyperglycemia. Insulin resistance impairs utilization of glucose by tissues. Ketoacidosis does not occur. Most common in older obese adults.
Latent autoimmune	Sometimes considered a subtype of type 1, results in slower destruction of pancreatic beta cells than with type 1 and positive autoantibodies (GABA). The patient may not need insulin for 2-4 years. Onset is at 30-50.

INSULIN AND CARBOHYDRATE METABOLISM AND CARBOHYDRATE DIGESTION

Carbohydrate digestion and metabolism begins when polysaccharides are converted to monosaccharides by digestive enzymes in the mouth and stomach, and the monosaccharides are then absorbed into the blood from the small intestine. The rise in glucose stimulates the pancreas to release proinsulin, which converts into insulin and moves glucose into the muscles and the liver, where glycogenesis, the process by which excess glucose is converted to glycogen for storage, occurs. Cells require insulin in order to use glucose for energy. The pancreas releases proinsulin (which is comprised of polypeptides A, B, and C) into the liver where the C-peptide is severed,

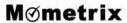

forming insulin. When blood glucose levels fall, the pancreas releases glucagon to stimulate the liver to convert glycogen back into glucose through glycogenolysis. If there are inadequate stores of glycogen (such as after fasting or with inadequate insulin levels), then the liver converts amino acids and lipids into glucose through gluconeogenesis.

GLUCOSE TOLERANCE TEST

A glucose tolerance test helps a physician understand and evaluate a patient's biological and chemical response to glucose. Glucose tolerance tests can be done with glucose administered to the patient either intravenously or orally. In a glucose tolerance test, blood glucose levels are taken at a fasting level, at one hour after glucose administration to the patient, at two hours after glucose administration, and again at three hours after glucose administration. Blood glucose levels can be taken at other times, as deemed necessary by the physician. The glucose tolerance test can be used to determine if a patient is diabetic, chemically speaking.

NORMAL GLUCOSE TOLERANCE CURVE AND GLUCOSE TOLERANCE CURVE OF A DIABETIC

A glucose tolerance curve of a non-diabetic patient shows a high blood glucose level at one hour after the administration of glucose, and the glucose level in the blood falls below the fasting glucose level at two hours after glucose administration. At three hours past glucose administration, the blood glucose levels in a non-diabetic patient should return to the fasting glucose level. The glucose tolerance curve of a diabetic patient will show above normal glucose levels, and glucose levels in the blood do not fall within the first two hours after glucose administration.

SERUM GLUCOSE ANALYSIS OF BLOOD

Glucose analysis of blood can be done with a glucometer, spectrophotometer, or manual methods, which include:

- Toluidine method: Measures glucose as a reducing substance and not as true glucose because other substances can also cause color reactions. Trichloroacetic acid (TCA) is used to precipitate proteins and then the sample is heated with glacial acetic acid, which causes the glucose in the filtrate to condense with Toluidine and change color (blue-green) with the level of glucose corresponding to the intensity of color. Toluidine is, however, carcinogenic.
- Enzymatic methods (glucose oxidase, glucose dehydrogenase, and hexokinase): These methods use a number of different reagents, solutions, and standards to bring about a color change that measures the amount of true glucose. These methods have been adapted for utilization in various types of glucose analyzers.
- Reagent strip: This quick screen method utilizes a drop of blood on a reagent strip, such as Dextrostix®, which changes color to show glucose concentration.

TESTS FOR CARBOHYDRATES, REDUCING SUBSTANCES, AND TESTS PERFORMED ON BLOOD, URINE, AND SPINAL FLUID

The most common **tests for carbohydrates** in the blood, urine, and spinal fluid are the glucose tests, but other forms of carbohydrates may be present. **Reducing substances** are carbohydrates that are present in a sample (such as blood, stool, urine, or spinal fluid) and help to diagnose a problem. For example, the presence of reducing substances in a stool specimen for a patient with diarrhea indicates that the diarrhea does not result from a parasitic or viral infection but rather an abnormality of carbohydrate excretion, such as lactase deficiency. Newborns are routinely screened for inborn errors of carbohydrate metabolism with reducing substance tests. If urine is negative for glucose but positive for reducing substances, then some other form of sugar (such as galactose, which indicates galactosemia) is present in the urine. Glucose is typically present in spinal fluid in lower amounts than in serum, and most reducing substances do not cross the blood-brain barrier.

USING SERUM OR PLASMA FOR GLUCOSE DETERMINATION

There are several reasons why the use of serum or plasma is preferred when determining glucose levels in the lab. For one, glucose is more stable in either plasma or serum than in whole blood. This is because any effects of glycolysis are lessened when whole blood is not used. Another reason is that when whole blood is used in glucose determination, the glucose values can vary with the varying hematocrit, thereby giving inaccurate results. Also, specificity for glucose is lower if whole blood is used as compared to the specificity if using serum or plasma. Finally, the presence of automated instruments in the laboratory makes it easier to use plasma or serum for glucose determination. This eliminates the need for mixing prior to sampling that would be required if whole blood were to be used.

GLYCOHEMOGLOBIN (A1C) PROCEDURE

Glycohemoglobin (A1C) test measures hemoglobin A with a glucose molecule (glycated/glycosylated hemoglobin). When levels of glucose in the blood increase, the glucose binds to hemoglobin in the red blood cells in amounts proportional to the circulating glucose. Since the average life span of a red blood cell is 120 days with cells continuously dying and being replaced, the A1C test provides an average glucose level over about the previous 3 months:

1. Normal value: 4% to 5.5%
2. Prediabetes: 5.7% to 6.4%

Elevation: ≥6.5%

Critical results: >6.9%

Testing is done on a whole venous blood sample collected in a tube with anticoagulant, such as EDTA, or a fingerstick capillary specimen. The specimen may be stored under refrigeration at 4° to 8°C if testing is not carried out immediately. A glycohemoglobin analyzer is used to obtain laboratory results.

PLASMA PROTEINS

Plasma proteins (albumin, alpha-1 globulin, alpha-2 globulin, beta globulin, gamma globulin, and fibrinogen) are synthesized in the liver, except for gamma globulin, which is synthesized in the reticuloendothelial system. All but fibrinogen are found in serum. Plasma proteins are converted into amino acids by proteases in the small intestines and the amino acids broken down through the processes of oxidative deamination or transamination to convert them to sugar to be used or stored by body cells for energy. Waste products of protein catabolism or excess plasma proteins are excreted in the urine. Because proteins act as acids, they help to maintain the pH level of the blood. Structure and function includes:

- Albumin: Comprised of 610 amino acids. Provides cell nutrition, transports of biomolecules (fatty acids, drugs), and maintains fluid balance.
- Alpha-1 globulin: Contains a number of complex proteins that include carbohydrates and lipids. Transports lipids.
- Alpha-2 globulin: Contains complex proteins, including plasminogen and prothrombin (which are necessary for coagulation) and ceruloplasmin (which is necessary for metabolism of copper).
- Beta globulin: Contains beta-lipoproteins and transferrin, which transports iron.

51

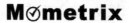

- <u>Gamma globulin</u>: These immunoglobulins (IgG, IgA, IgD, IgE, and IgM) are antibodies that are part of the body's immune response.
- <u>Fibrinogen</u>: Fibrous protein that contains enzymes (alkaline phosphatase, acid phosphatase) and promotes coagulation.

GLOBULINS AND IMMUNOGLOBULINS

Globulins: A class of proteins that has a spherical or globular shape that is found in blood plasma. They are produced by the liver. Globulins, unlike albumin, are insoluble in water and in a half-saturated ammonium solution. They can also be coagulated with the addition of heat. Globulins are subdivided into various classes, alpha 1, alpha 2, beta, and gamma on the basis of their mobility at an alkaline pH of 8.6 when analyzed through electrophoresis techniques.

Immunoglobulins: A type of globulin that is produced by lymphoid cells in the human body. They serve as antibodies in the human immune system. They are divided up into 5 types based on structure: IgA, IgD, IgE, IgG, and IgM. IgG is the most common immunoglobulin, constituting 70% of the immunoglobulins found in blood.

ALBUMIN

Albumin is a protein that is produced in the liver, and it is the most abundant protein found in human serum. It constitutes approximately 55% of plasma proteins. Albumin can be coagulated with the addition of heat. Albumin is soluble in water, as well as in a half-saturated ammonium sulfate solution. Furthermore, albumin plays a large part in osmotic regulation in the blood and in fatty acid transport in the body. Albumin can be found in many body tissues.

DENATURATION

Denaturation is a process that modifies and alters a protein's tertiary structure. The tertiary structure of a protein is the high order structure of the protein, and it describes the structure of the protein when the protein is in its folded and globular form. The process of denaturation involves the breaking of the bonds in a protein. The bonds can be covalent, disulfide, or hydrogen bonds. Denaturation can be caused by extreme heat, agitation or shaking of the protein, or chemical treatment of the protein with detergents, acids, organic solvents (such as alcohol), or salts. When a protein is denatured, some of the properties of the protein can be lost. For example, the protein can become less soluble. Also, enzymes can lose their catalytic function when they are denatured.

PRINCIPLES OF SERUM PROTEIN ELECTROPHORESIS AND PROTEIN ANALYSIS

Total protein is measured with spectrophotometry and fractions of different plasma proteins by **serum protein electrophoresis** combined with immunoprecipitation (immunofixation electrophoresis, which divides the proteins according to size and charge). Plasma proteins include:

Total protein	0-5 days: 3.8-6.2 g/dL.	<u>Increased</u>: dehydration, monoclonal/polyclonal gammopathies, myeloma, sarcoidosis, chronic hepatic disease, leprosy, Waldenström macroglobulinemia.
	Adult: 6-8 g/dL.	<u>Decreased</u>: Hypervolemia, burns, chronic alcoholism, liver disorders, kidney disorders, CHF, hyperthyroidism, malabsorption syndromes, neoplasms, pregnancy, starvation, prolonged immobilization.
Albumin	3.4-4.8 g/dL	<u>Increased</u>: Dehydration, diarrhea, vomiting.
	55.5%	<u>Decreased</u>: Renal disease, malnutrition, severe burns.

Alpha-1 globulin	0.2-0.4 g/dL	Increased: Acute/chronic inflammatory diseases
	5.3%	Decreased: Hereditary disease.
Alpha-2 globulin	0.4-0.8 g/dL	Increased: Diabetes, pancreatitis, hemolysis.
	8.6%	Decreased: Nephrotic syndrome, malignancies, inflammation, severe burn recovery period.
Beta globulin	0.5-1.0 g/dL	Increased: Hyperlipoproteinemias, monoclonal gammopathies.
	13.4%	Decreased: Hypo-β-lipoproteinemia, IgA deficiency.
Gamma globulin	0.6-1.2 g/dL	Increased: Hepatic disease, chronic infections, autoimmune disorders, and lymphoproliferative disorders, multiple myeloma.
	11%	Decreased: Immune deficiency/suppression.
	IgG—80%	Note gamma globulin consists of 5 bands of immunoglobulins on electrophoresis: IgG, IgA, IgM, IgD, and IgE.
	IgA—15%	
	IgM—5%	
	IgD—0.2%	
	IgE—Trace.	

PURPOSE OF AN AFP TEST ON A PREGNANT WOMAN

AFP stands for alpha-fetoprotein, and it is a protein that is produced by a fetus' liver. Alpha-fetoprotein can be detected in the mother's blood through a blood test. AFP reaches its highest concentration in the mother's blood between 12 and 15 weeks of gestation. Drawing the mother's blood at this time will thereby give the peak AFP released by the fetus. If the AFP levels in the mother's blood are found to be unusually high, there may be medical problems with the fetus, such as neural tube defects, including spina bifida, and anencephaly, or kidney problems. High AFP levels can also indicate twins. If the AFP levels are found to be unusually low, Down syndrome may be indicated. Ultrasound and amniocentesis can be used to confirm the results. Through amniocentesis, a sample of the amniotic fluid can be retrieved, and the AFP in the amniotic fluid can then be determined. Radioimmunoassay or immunoprecipitin methods can be used to quantify the amount of AFP present.

BIURET PROCEDURE AND QUANTIFYING TOTAL PROTEINS IN A SERUM

The biuret procedure is used to determine the amount of protein in a sample. The procedure depends on the reaction between peptide linkages in the protein and copper ions in an alkaline solution. A reddish/violet color indicates the presence of peptide linkages, or proteins. The biuret procedure gives an accurate quantitation of the amount of total proteins found in a serum. A larger amount of proteins in a serum will have a larger quantity of peptide bonds, since all amino acids of proteins are joined by peptide bonds. A larger quantity of peptide bonds will lead to a more intense color produced by the reaction with the copper ions the biuret procedure. Typically, 4-6 peptide linkages will react/join with one copper ion complex. However, with a minimum of 2 peptide linkages available, the reaction will work, forming a reddish/violet colored product. Therefore, a tripeptide is the smallest protein that will react in the biuret procedure.

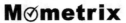

KJELDAHL TECHNIQUE FOR DETERMINING TOTAL PROTEIN IN A SERUM

The Kjeldahl technique is the reference method for quantifying the total protein found in a serum sample. The basis of the technique is the quantification of the number of peptide bonds present in the protein in the serum. In other words, the nitrogen content of the protein present is quantified. Through a reaction with sulfuric acid, the protein present undergoes digestion, which converts the nitrogen present in the protein to ammonium ions. The ammonium ion can then undergo distillation, which will give off ammonia, which can then be titrated. Or, the ammonium ion produced can be mixed with Nessler's reagent, which will form a colored product. This colored product can then be read spectrophotometrically. The Kjeldahl technique is thought to be too cumbersome to be used on a routine basis in the laboratory, but it is still considered to be the reference method for quantifying the total protein in a serum.

ENZYME

An enzyme is a protein that is produced by living cells that consists of one or more polypeptide chains. These specific kinds of proteins are proteins that serve as catalysts for biochemical reactions that take place in the human body. Enzymes catalyze reactions by reducing the activation energy that is needed for that particular reaction to occur. In doing so, the enzyme does not change its own function or structure. Like any protein, enzymes can be denatured due to a variety of reasons, including excessive heat, agitation, or pH changes, and this denaturation can lead to a loss of catalyzing ability (activity) of the enzyme. When the enzyme becomes denatured, the 3D shape of its polypeptide chain is altered, therefore changing the activity of the enzyme. There are 6 main classes of enzymes: Hydrolases, isomerases, ligases, lyases, oxidoreductases, and transferases.

CLASSES OF ENZYMES

Ligases: Ligases are enzymes that catalyze a reaction that results in the covalent bonding of 2 separate molecules. This bonding is accompanied by the hydrolysis of ATP. An example of a ligase is glutamine synthetase.

Lyases: Lyases are enzymes that catalyze the cleavage of molecules between their carbon-to-carbon bonds. Lyases catalyze these reactions without the addition of water. An example of a lyase is aldolase.

Oxidoreductases: Oxidoreductases are enzymes that catalyze reactions dealing with the transfer of electrons (hydrogen atoms). They are important enzymes in respiration and in the production of energy in the human body. An example of an oxidoreductase is lactate dehydrogenase.

Hydrolases: Hydrolases are enzymes that catalyze the hydrolysis of certain molecules, such as nucleic acids, proteins, and fats. Hydrolysis is the splitting of molecules by adding water to them. An example of a hydrolase is amylase.

Isomerases: Isomerases are enzymes that catalyze intramolecular conversion in molecules. An example of an isomerase is glucose phosphate isomerase.

Transferases: Transferases are enzymes that catalyze reactions that deal with the transfer of a chemical group between molecules. Some transferases catalyze the transfer of amino groups, and these are called transaminases. Transferases can also transfer methyl (transmethylases) and phosphate groups (kinases), in addition to others.

EFFECT OF TEMPERATURE OR pH ON ENZYME ASSAYS

Every enzyme has an optimal temperature and pH that will allow for the highest level of enzymatic activity of that enzyme. Therefore, enzyme assays are affected by the temperature and pH at which

54

they are performed. If the temperature or pH is lower than the optimal values, the enzyme's catalytic ability (activity) will be lower than what would be expected. However, if the temperature or pH is higher than the optimal values, rate of the reactions will increase. A 10 degree Celsius increase in temperature will usually lead to a twofold increase in reaction rates. However, it should be noted that enzymes, like other proteins, can denature at high temperatures or extreme pH levels. If this happens, the enzyme can lose its preferred structure, which would lower the enzyme's catalytic ability.

ISOENZYMES/ENZYMES

Lipase	0-6 units/L	Pancreatic digestive enzyme involved in fat digestion.
		Obtain 1 mL specimen in red or tiger capped tube or green topped heparin tube for enzymatic spectrophotometry.
		Increased: Pancreatic disease, renal failure, and acute cholecystitis.
Amylase	30-110 units/L.	Pancreatic (and parotid) digestive enzyme splits starch into disaccharides. Obtain 1 mL specimen in red or tiger capped tube or green topped heparin tube for enzymatic spectrophotometry. Increased: Conditions that involve cellular destruction, acuter appendicitis, abdominal trauma, alcoholism, bile tract disease/obstruction, burns, pancreatic cancer, pancreatitis, peritonitis.
		Decreased: Advanced liver disease, pancreatic insufficiency, pancreatectomy.
C-reactive protein	Conventional assay: 0-0.8 mg/dL.	Produced by the liver in response to an inflammatory response that causes neutrophils, granulocytes and macrophages to secrete cytokines. Obtain 1 mL sample in red or tiger-capped tube for nephelometry.
	Immunoassay: Low risk <1 mg/dL High >10 mg/dL	Increased: Inflammatory conditions, IBD, MI, SLE, rheumatic fever, pregnancy (last half), RA.
Ceruloplas min (CP)	10-54 mg/dL	Copper-carrying enzyme. Obtain 1 mL sample in red or tiger-capped tube for nephelometry.
		Increased: inflammatory conditions, leukemia, copper intoxication, various cancers, RA, Hodgkin disease.
		Decreased: Menkes disease, Wilson disease. Copper insufficiency.

Ge

ELEVATED SERUM ENZYME LEVELS EXAMPLES

1. An elevated serum level of **aldolase** is implicated in many muscular disorders, such as muscular dystrophy. It is also elevated in patients with myocardial infarctions (heart attacks), toxic acute hepatitis, viral hepatitis, and megaloblastic anemia.
2. An elevated level of serum **amylase** is often associated with acute pancreatitis.
3. An elevated serum level of **creatine kinase** is usually caused by damage to brain tissue, as in cerebrovascular accidents (strokes), damage to cardiac muscle, as in myocardial infarctions (heart attacks), or damage to skeletal muscle. Elevated serum creatine kinase can also be associated with hypothyroidism.
4. Elevated serum levels of both **alanine aminotransferase** and **aspartate aminotransferase** are often indicative of acute hepatitis.
5. An elevated serum level of **alkaline phosphatase** can be associated with Paget's disease (osteitis deformans).

CARDIAC BIOMARKERS

When the heart is damaged, it releases **cardiac biomarkers**, which include:

- Creatine kinase (CK) isoenzyme (MB): Specific to heart muscle. Increases within 4-8 hours of a heart attack, peaks at about 24 hours (earlier with thrombolytic therapy) and remains elevated for 72 hours. (Values: electrophoresis 4%, immunoassay 0-3 ng/mL, index 0-2.5)
- Myoglobin (heme protein that transports oxygen): Found in skeletal and cardiac muscles. Level increases 1-3 hours after a heart attack and peak within 12 hours. While increase is not specific to MI, failure to increase can rule out an MI. (Values: Male 28-72 ng/mL, female 25-58 ng/mL)
- Troponin I: Found only in the heart muscle. Levels increase 3-6 hours after heart attack, peak in 14-20 hours, and return to normal within 5-7 days. (Values: <0.05 ng/mL)
- Troponin T: Found in heart and skeletal muscle. Levels increase 3-6 hours after heart attack, peak in 12-24 hours, and return to normal in 10-15 days. (Values: <0.2 ng/mL)
- Brain Natriuretic Peptide (BNP): Substance secreted by the ventricular muscle with increased volume and pressure. Increased level indicates heart failure. (Values: 0-74 years <125 pg/mL, >75 years <449 pg/mL)
- Lactate dehydrogenase (LDH): Released from damaged cells in organs and other tissues. Increases with acute MI, anemias, conditions with platelet destruction, liver disease, and musculoskeletal damage. Peaks in 72 hours of MI and returns to normal in 10-14 days. (15-43 years: 90-156 units/L, >43 years: 90-176 units/L)

PRINCIPLES OF ISOENZYME ELECTROPHORESIS AND HEMOGLOBIN ELECTROPHORESIS

Isoenzyme electrophoresis separates enzymes into components with different molecular structure (isoenzymes) according to size and charge. For example lactase dehydrogenase (LDH) has 5 isoenzymes, numbered consecutively, but LDH1 is found in the heart muscle and increases with an MI while LDH5 increases with liver disease. Creatine kinase has three isoenzymes: CK-BB in brain and lungs, CK-MG in cardiac muscle, and CK-MM in skeletal muscle. Alkaline phosphatase has

12 isoenzymes, including the bone, liver and the liver fractions, which are most important for diagnoses.

Hemoglobin electrophoresis		
Hemoglobin (identifies normal and abnormal forms of Hgb)	Hgb A >95%	Most common form of Hgb.
	Hgb A2 1.5-3.7%	Increased: Hyperthyroidism, sickle cell trait, and β-thalassemia and megaloblastic anemia. Decreased: Iron deficiency anemia, sideroblastic anemia, erythroleukemia.
	Hgb F (fetal): Newborn—70-77%, 6 mo—3-7%. Adult—<2%	Increased: Aplastic anemia, anemia of blood loss, leukemia, myeloproliferative disorders, pernicious anemia, thalassemias, sickle cell disease.
	Hgb D, E, H, S, C Presence indicates abnormality	Found in inherited hemoglobinopathies. Increased E: thalassemia-like disorder. Increased: Sickle cell disease. Increased H: α-thalassemia.

ENDOCRINOLOGY CONCEPTS

The **endocrine system** includes numerous glands that have secretory cells but no ducts, so hormones produced are absorbed into the vascular system. Many hormones function under a negative feedback system: When the hormone level decreases, production increases, and when the hormone level increases, production is inhibited. Positive feedback occurs when the activity in an organ that is outside normal triggers release of hormone, such as increased release of oxytocin during childbirth and decrease in oxytocin after childbirth. Complex feedback involves interactions among a number of hormones, such as occurs with regulation of thyroid hormones. Some hormones are affected by nervous system reactions, such as when fear or anger triggers release of epinephrine. Some hormones cause the release of other hormones, such as thyrotropin-releasing hormone and prolactin-releasing hormone, while others inhibit hormones, such as prolactin-inhibiting hormone and somatostatin.

STEPS IN THE PRODUCTION OF HORMONES IN THE THYROID

The first step that needs to take place in order for the thyroid to produce its various hormones is for the thyroid to capture iodine from the rest of the body. Iodine can be captured from the gastrointestinal tract, for example. Once the thyroid has captured iodine, the iodine must then be activated. The activated form of iodine is called organic iodine. The organic, activated iodine then undergoes a process called organification. Organification is the process in which the iodine is attached to the tyrosine residues that are part of the protein thyroglobulin (TG). Thyroid stimulating hormone (TSH) then helps separate the iodinated tyrosines (the iodine coupled with the tyrosine) form the thyroglobulins. This forms T_3 (triiodothyroxine) and T_4 (thyroxine), and these hormones are then released into the bloodstream. This separation and creation of triiodothyroxine and thyroxine occurs on an as-needed basis in the body, regulated by TSH.

PREGNANCY HORMONES

LUTEINIZING HORMONE (LH) AND HUMAN PLACENTAL LACTOGEN (HPL)

Luteinizing Hormone (LH): Luteinizing hormone is a hormone that is released only by the pituitary gland. LH helps to stimulate the release of an egg (ovulation), and it also helps stimulate the release of progesterone by the corpus luteum after ovulation. Luteinizing hormone also plays an important role in helping prepare the uterine wall for a fertilized egg to successfully implant.

Human Placental Lactogen (HPL): HPL is a protein hormone that is secreted and created only by the placenta of a pregnant woman. HPL plays an important role in making sure that a fetus receives the necessary energy that it needs to thrive during pregnancy. HPL accomplishes this by affect the mother's metabolism during pregnancy. HPL is measurable in the mother's blood between the 7th and 9th weeks of pregnancy, and it reaches its maximum values near the end of the pregnancy.

PROGESTERONE AND HUMAN CHORIONIC GONADOTROPIN (HCG)

Progesterone: Progesterone is a steroid hormone that is necessary to successfully maintain a pregnancy. After a woman ovulates, the level of progesterone in her blood increases dramatically. The progesterone helps prepare the uterine wall for a fertilized egg to implant, in the case of a pregnancy. The high levels of progesterone also help prevent an early spontaneous miscarriage of the pregnancy. During pregnancy, the main source of progesterone is the placenta. Progesterone also helps in the production of milk in the woman's mammary glands.

Human Chorionic Gonadotropin (hCG): hCG is a protein hormone that is released by the placenta. hCG is released very soon after conception during a pregnancy, and it is the hormone that is often tested for with a home pregnancy test to determine the existence of a pregnancy. The level of hCG in a woman's blood is at its highest level during the first trimester of pregnancy. It drops off after that, so that a woman in her seventh month may test negative for pregnancy.

DETERMINING OVULATION WITH PROGESTERONE LEVEL IN BLOOD PLASMA

A woman's menstrual cycle consists of two phases. The first phase, which is the phase from the first day of menstruation through ovulation (the release of an egg from the woman's ovary) is called the follicular stage. In this particular stage, progesterone tends to be low (less than 2 ng/mL). After a woman has ovulated, the luteal phase begins. The luteal phase is considered to be the day after ovulation up through the day before the start of menstruation. If a woman has ovulated, the progesterone level in her blood plasma should be higher than it was in the luteal phase, usually higher than 5 ng/mL. Progesterone production by the corpus luteum rises sharply after ovulation, therefore, the higher level of progesterone in the blood plasma indicates ovulation already took place. If the progesterone level does not increase during the second half of the cycle, a woman has not ovulated, and she will be having what is called an anovulatory cycle.

EFFECT OF VITAMIN D AND PARATHYROID HORMONE (PTH) ON PLASMA CALCIUM LEVELS

Vitamin D: When Vitamin D is hydroxylized (the addition of an OH group to the Vitamin D), a compound is produced that increases the absorption of phosphates and calcium in the intestines.

Parathyroid Hormone (PTH): Parathyroid hormone is a hormone that helps maintain calcium levels in plasma. It helps move calcium from bones into the blood. PTH increases the creation of a particular derivative of Vitamin D, which causes an increase in the absorption of calcium in the intestines, and an increase in bone resorption. PTH production is shut off when normal calcium levels in the plasma are restored. PTH also helps regulate the amount of phosphorus.

EFFECT OF PLASMA PHOSPHATES ON PLASMA CALCIUM LEVELS

Plasma Phosphates: Inorganic plasma phosphates and plasma calcium have an inverse relationship. An increase in plasma phosphates will result in a decrease in plasma calcium.

Calcitonin: Calcitonin is a hormone that is produced by the thyroid gland in humans. It helps regulate the metabolism of calcium. If there are elevated levels of calcium in plasma, the thyroid gland secretes calcitonin. The calcitonin then prevents the bones from reabsorbing calcium, slows down the destruction of bone, and minimizes the amount of calcium released into the blood.

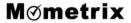

LEVELS OF DYSFUNCTION RELATING TO ENDOCRINE PROBLEMS

There are three levels of dysfunction when discussing endocrine problems: Primary, secondary, and tertiary. The primary level of dysfunction refers to a problem within the particular gland where the hormone in question is produced. For example, this could be a direct problem with the ovaries, which secrete estrogen. The secondary level of dysfunction refers to a problem with the pituitary gland in the brain. In this case, the pituitary gland releases luteinizing hormone (LH) that tells the ovary to give off estrogen. Lack of pituitary LH prevents the release of estrogen from the ovaries, since estrogen release is regulated by LH. Finally, the tertiary level of dysfunction refers to a problem in the hypothalamus in the brain. The hypothalamus creates releasing factors, which then affect the hormone production in the pituitary gland, and the ovaries in turn.

ADDISON'S DISEASE

Addison's disease is characterized by insufficient adrenal gland function. This can lead to anemia, weakness, low blood pressure, and brownish/bronze pigmentation of the skin and mucous membranes. The adrenal glands of a patient with Addison's disease do not produce sufficient adrenal hormones, such as aldosterone and cortisol. The decreased production of aldosterone can affect extracellular fluid volume in the individual, as well as the body's overall electrolyte balance. This occurs when the decreased amount of sodium reabsorption by the renal tubules leads to decreased water retention and the decreased production of chloride. This decreased water retention and chloride production will then lead to a decrease in extracellular fluid volume in the patient. Furthermore, the decreased sodium reabsorption will interfere with the production of hydrogen and potassium ions in the renal tubules. This will lead to an increase in the hydrogen and potassium ion concentrations in serum.

CUSHING'S SYNDROME

Cushing's Syndrome is a disorder that is often related to an abnormal (increased) production of cortisol by the adrenal glands. Patients with Cushing's Syndrome usually have an tumor in their pituitary gland or a problem with their adrenal glands. This leads to a problem with the regulation of the hormone ACTH, adrenocorticotropic hormone. This abnormal production of ACTH is what leads to the abnormality in the cortisol production. People with Cushing's Syndrome can suffer from obesity, weak muscles, and fatigue. They are also at a higher risk of developing heart disease, diabetes, or high blood pressure later in life. There is also a higher level of 17-ketosteroids found in the urine of someone with Cushing's Syndrome.

HORMONE TESTS

Adrenocorticotropic hormone (ACTH)	ACTH: 10-18 years: 6-55 pg/mL >18 years: 6-58 pg/mL	ACTH is produced in the anterior pituitary gland and released in response to increased hypothalamic-releasing factor. ACTH stimulates increased production of glucocorticoids (cortisol), androgens, and mineralocorticoids by the adrenals. ACTH is part of the hypothalamic-pituitary-adrenal axis. <u>Increased</u>: Addison disease (with low cortisol), Cushing disease (with high cortisol), carcinoid syndrome, congenital adrenal hyperplasia, depression, Nelson syndrome, septic shock/sepsis. <u>Decreased</u>: Adrenal adenoma or cancer, Cushing syndrome, steroid therapy.
	<u>Stimulation with cosyntropin</u>: Cortisol 18-20 mcg/dL or cortisol level increases 7 mcg/dL over baseline <u>Stimulation with metyrapone</u> (overnight): Cortisol <2 mcg/dL next day; ACTH >75 pg/mL	
	ACTH suppression with dexamethasone (overnight): Cortisol <1.87 mcg/dL next day	
Cortisol	<u>8AM</u>: 12-18 years—10-280 mcg/dL; >18 years—5-25 mcg/dL.	Primary glucocorticoid secreted by adrenal glands. Stimulates gluconeogenesis, serves as insulin antagonist, suppresses inflammatory response, and mobilizes proteins and fats. Test measures adrenal function.
	<u>4 PM</u>: 12-18 years—10-272 mcg/dL; >18 years—3-16 mcg/dL	
Antidiuretic hormone (ADH)	ADH: 0-18 years 0.5-1.5 pg/mL	Produced in hypothalamus, stored in posterior pituitary gland, and released with decreased blood volume or increased serum osmolality. Causes the kidneys to reabsorb more water to maintain proper osmolality and fluid balance. <u>Increased</u>: Brain tumor, CNS disorders, hypovolemia, Guillain-Barré, diabetes insipidus (DI) (nephrogenic), SIADH. <u>Decreased</u>: Hypervolemia, nephrotic syndrome, DI (pituitary), pituitary surgery, psychogenic polydipsia.
	>18 years 0-5 pg/mL	
	Correlated with serum osmolality: 270-280 mOsm/kg—<1.5 pg/mL 280-285 mOsm/kg—<2.5 pg/mL 285-290 mOsm/kg—1-5 pg/mL 290-295 mOsm/kg—2-7 pg/mL 295-300 mOsm/kg—4-12 pg/mL	

60

Aldosterone	Aldosterone: 11-15 years supine 2-22 ng/dL 11-15 years upright 4-48 ng/dL >15 years supine 3-16 ng/dL >15 years upright 7-30 ng/dL	Mineralocorticoid produced by adrenal glands in response to increased potassium, decreased sodium, or decreased blood volume. Release triggered by angiotensin II. Helps to regulate sodium and potassium levels. Increased: Adenomas (with decreased renin), cardiac failure, COPD, cirrhosis, diuretic/laxative abuse, hypovolemia, nephrotic syndrome, starvation, toxemia. Decreased: (With hypertension) Addison disease; (Without hypertension) alcohol intoxication, diabetes, Turner syndrome.
Dehydroepiandrosterone sulfate (DHEAS)	Varies by age, gender, and Tanner stage: Male: 3-6 years—0-50 mcg/dL, 15-19 years—88-483 mcg/dL, 20-29 years—280-640 mcg/dL, 60-69 years—42-290 mcg/dL Female: 3-6 years—0-50 mcg/dL, 15-19 years—63-373 mcg/dL, 20-29 years—65-380 mcg/dL, 60-69 years—13-130 mcg/dL	Metabolite of primary adrenal androgen (DHEA), synthesized in adrenals and testes. Can convert into testosterone or estradiol. Increased: Cushing syndrome, anovulation, hirsutism, polycystic ovarian syndrome, adrenal tumors (virilizing), ACTH-producing tumors. Decreased: Addison disease, hyperlipidemia, pregnancy, psoriasis, psychosis.
Parathyroid hormone (PTH)	2-20 years: 9-52 pg/mL >20 years: 10-065 pg/mL	Produced in parathyroid glands and released in response to low calcium levels to mobilize movement of calcium from bones into blood. Increased: Hyperparathyroidism, fluorosis, Zollinger-Ellison syndrome, pseudogout. Decreased: Hypoparathyroidism, hyperparathyroidism (associated with increased serum calcium), sarcoidosis.

THYROID FUNCTION TESTS

Thyroid-stimulating hormone (TSH)	0.4-6.15 μ/U/mL	Released from pituitary gland, triggered by thyrotropin-releasing hormone (hypothalamus). Stimulates thyroid to produce triiodothyronine (T3) and thyroxine (T4), which regulate metabolism. Increased: Hypothyroidism. Decreased: Hyperthyroidism.
Free T3	17-20 ng/dL	Regulates cell metabolic rate, cell growth, and cell differentiation. Increased: Hyperthyroidism, high altitude, T3 toxicosis. Decreased: Hypothyroidism, malnutrition, chronic disease (non-thyroid), late pregnancy.
T3 resin uptake	25-35%	Test to estimate amounts of free T3, T4, and TBG. Increased: Hyperthyroidism. Decreased: Hypothyroidism.
T4 total	4.5-11.5 μg/dL	May be affected by levels of TBG. Increased: Iodine toxicity, psychiatric disorder, hepatitis, hyperthyroidism, obesity, thyrotoxicosis (Graves') and thyrotoxicosis factitia. Decreased: Low TBG level, hypothyroidism, panhypopituitarism, excessive exercise.
Free T4	0.9-1.7 ng/dL	Precursor to T3, not affected by levels of TBG. Increased: Hyperthyroidism. Decreased: Hypothyroidism.
Thyroxine-binding globulin (TBG)	0-50 ng/mL	Protein that transports thyroid hormones. Increased: Thyroid cancer, Graves diseases, thyroiditis, thyrotoxicosis. Decreased: Thyrotoxicosis factitia, administration of thyroid hormones, and congenital athyrosis (in neonates).

24-HOUR URINE ENDOCRINOLOGY TESTS

Thyroid hormone test	T3: 15-18 years 1.1-2.7 nmol/L	Urine levels may be higher than serum because serum levels vary during the day.
	>18 years 0.9-2.4 nmol/L	
	T4: 14-17 years 5-9.8 mcg/dL	Urine levels may be higher than serum.
	≥18 years 4.8-10.4 mcg/dL	
	Selenium ≤200 mcg/L with creatinine correction <25 mcg/g	Selenium converts T4 into T3. Levels may be higher or lower with cancer. Levels are decreased in children, older adults, and pregnant women.
5-Hydroxyin doleacetic acid (5-HIAA)	2-10 years <8 mg/g creatinine	Product of serotonin metabolism. Used to measure serotonin level. Increased: carcinoid and neuroendocrine tumors, cystic fibrosis, celiac disease. Decreased: renal disease, phenylketonuria
	>10 years <6 mg/d	

REPRODUCTIVE HORMONE TESTS

Follicle-stimulating hormone (FSH)	Male: 1.4-15.5 IU/mL.	Used to manage/diagnose menstrual problems, infertility, abnormal sexual development. Increased: Alcoholism, Klinefelter syndrome, hypogonadism, Turner syndrome, precocious puberty. Decreased: Anorexia nervosa, hemochromatosis, polycystic ovary disease, pregnancy, sickle cell anemia, hypothalamic disorder.
	Female: Varies according to cycle, increases during ovulation: 7.2-17.2 IU/mL.	
	Postmenopausal: 19-100 IU/mL.	
Luteinizing hormone (LH)	Male; 0.5-1.9 IU/mL.	Used to assess gonadal function, fertility issues, treatment response. Increased: Gonadal disorders, menopause. Decreased: Anorexia nervosa, malnutrition, hypothalamic/pituitary dysfunction, stress.
	Female, varies according to cycle, increases during ovulation: 21.9-80.	
	Postmenopausal: 14.2-52.3 IU/mL.	
17-ketosteroids	Varies widely according to age, gender, and Tanner stage	Used to evaluate androgen excess, adrenal tumors, congenital adrenal hyperplasia, and (in females) infertility, amenorrhea, and excess hair growth. Increased: Cushing syndrome, polycystic ovary syndrome, hirsutism, anovulation. Decreased: Addison disease, adrenal insufficiency, hyperlipidemia, pregnancy, psoriasis, psychosis.
Estrogen (estriol, estradiol, and estrone)	Estriol: Levels vary	Measured during pregnancy, evident by 9 weeks.
	Estradiol: Levels vary by gender, age, menstrual cycle, and menopause	Used to diagnose infertility associated with tumor or ovarian failure.
	Estrone—primary source of estrogen after menopause. Males: 10-60 pg/mL Adult females: 17-200 pg/mL Postmenopausal females: 7-40 pg/mL.	Estrone—used to assess estrogen level in post-menopausal women and to assess estrogen levels in males and females with ovarian, testicular, and adrenal malignancies.

| **Testosterone** | Varies by age and gender:
Male 8-10 y: 0-25 ng/dL
Male 13-15 y: 15-500 ng/dL
Male >15 y: 241-827 ng/dL
Female 8-10 y: 0-30 ng/dL
Female 13-15 y: 0-50 ng/dL
Female >15 y: 15-70 ng/dL | Used to assess disorders of puberty and infertility and gonadal/adrenal function. <u>Increased</u>: Adrenal hyperplasia, adrenocortical tumors, hirsutism, hyperthyroidism, idiopathic sexual precocity, polycystic ovaries, testicular tumors, virilizing ovarian tumors. <u>Decreased</u>: Anovulation, cryptorchidism, alcoholism, impotence, Klinefelter syndrome, myotonic dystrophy, hypogonadism, hypopituitarism, uremia. |

DETERMINING THE INORGANIC PHOSPHATE CONCENTRATION IN A SERUM

The basis of this determination is reacting a deproteinized serum with a molybdate reagent. The phosphate in the serum, once reacting with the molybdate reagent, will form a phosphomolybdate compound. This compound can then be combined with a reducing agent to form molybdenum blue. The resulting molybdenum blue can then be measured in the laboratory spectrophotometrically to determine the inorganic phosphate concentration in the serum.

LIPOPROTEIN COMPLEX AND METABOLISM OF CHOLESTEROL AND TRIGLYCERIDES

Lipoproteins are complex proteins that transport lipids (fats), such as triglycerides and cholesterol (which are insoluble in water) in fluids (extracellular fluids and blood) between body tissues, especially between the liver and adipose tissue, with the protein wrapping around the lipids. Cholesterol is obtained from the diet as well as through biosynthesis within the liver and intestines through a number of steps that convert Acetyl-CoA into cholesterol. Cholesterol is used for steroid and bile synthesis. A number of different lipoproteins are involved in transport with different proteins in their outer layer: chylomicrons, very low density (VLD), intermediate density (IDL), low density (LDL), and high density (HDL). Chylomicrons and VDL carry triglycerides to the cells. LDL carries cholesterol to cells, HDL carries excess cholesterol away from cells to the liver where it is oxidized and secreted in bile or converted into bile salts. When glucose stores are low, glucagon triggers release of lipase, which along with bile breaks down triglycerides through lipolysis in the intestine to release fatty acids and glycerol, which can be converted to glucose.

APOLIPOPROTEINS AND DETERMINING THE QUANTITY OF APOLIPOPROTEINS

An apolipoprotein is a protein that when combined with a lipid forms a lipoprotein. There are 5 major types of apolipoproteins, A, B, C, D, and E. In addition, there are at least 12 different forms of apolipoproteins as well. Some of the methods that can be used to determine the quantity of apolipoproteins in a sample are: radioimmunoassay (RIA), immunonephelometry (INA), enzyme-linked immunoassay (ELISA), electroimmunoassay (EIA), radial immunodiffusion (RID), and fluorescence immunoassay (FIA).

NONESTERIFIED FATTY ACIDS

Nonesterified fatty acids are also known as free fatty acids. Free fatty acids are fatty acids that can bind to other molecules. When they are not bound to other molecules, they are called free fatty acids. Nonesterified fatty acids (NEFA) make up a very small part of the lipids present in plasma, and the albumin in plasma is what transports these fatty acids when they are not bound to other molecules. In determining the amount of nonesterified fatty acids in a sample, titration is often used. The reagents that are used are thymol blue and sodium hydroxide solutions. Either

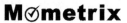

heparinized plasma or a serum can be used for the analysis. Also, the analysis should be completed as soon as possible after drawing the blood from the patient to avoid lipolysis, which would contribute to inaccurate results.

PROSTAGLANDINS AND THEIR EFFECTS ON THE HUMAN BODY

Prostaglandins are part of a group of lipid compounds that are derived from essential fatty acids. Prostaglandins are hormone- like substances produced by cell membranes as needed throughout the body. Prostaglandins have many effects on the human body. They can stimulate the contraction of the uterus, thereby inducing labor in a pregnant woman. They can help defend against infection, regulate metabolism, inhibit the aggregation of platelets, and control blood pressure. They also play a part in the contraction of the body's smooth muscle and gastrointestinal tract. They also play a part in inflammation in the body and they can help transmit nerve impulses as well.

TOTAL ANION CONTENT OF SERUM BY CONCENTRATION IN A HEALTHY ADULT

The highest concentration of the total anion content of a serum is of chloride, followed by bicarbonate. The next highest concentration is that of negatively charged proteins. These proteins make up approximately 16 mmol of charge per liter. Lactate has the next highest concentration, and finally, ketone bodies, such as acetate, make up the smallest concentration of the total anion content of a serum.

WATER-SOLUBLE VITAMINS AND FAT-SOLUBLE VITAMINS

Thiamin, ascorbic acid, niacin, and riboflavin are all water-soluble vitamins. Vitamin A, Vitamin D, Vitamin E, and vitamin K are all fat soluble.

SCURVY

Scurvy is a disease due to a deficiency in ascorbic acid (Vitamin C). Unlike most other animals, humans cannot create Vitamin C on their own -- Vitamin C needs to be ingested in the foods that humans eat (or through vitamin supplements). Patients with scurvy often have bleeding and puffy gums, loose teeth, body weakness, and trouble with wounds healing properly. They also can have excessive bleeding throughout their bodies. Consuming a diet high in Vitamin C can help prevent scurvy. High sources of Vitamin C include: Oranges, lemons, limes, grapefruits, broccoli, collards, strawberries, and brussel sprouts. In the United States, most cases of scurvy are found among children between the ages of 7 months and 2 years.

BERIBERI

Beriberi is a disease that is due to a deficiency in Vitamin B_1 (thiamin). Beriberi can cause fatigue, digestive problems, edema, emotional lability and other cardiovascular and nervous system problems. Beriberi is rare in developed countries, such as the United States, but is epidemic in Asia, where white rice is the staple diet. In the United States, beriberi is most often seen in the elderly (tea and toast diet) and in alcoholics. A diet that includes unbleached cereals, green vegetables, meat or legumes, and fruit or thiamin hydrochloride supplementation can cure beriberi. However, if not treated, beriberi can be a fatal disease.

NEWBORN BABIES AND VITAMIN K SHOT

Vitamin K is a very important vitamin because it is related to proper clotting of the blood. It helps form prothrombin to make a clot. If there is a lack of Vitamin K, there will be a corresponding decrease in the production of prothrombin. Adults with decreased prothrombin have increased PT/PTT times, broken capillaries and bruising. Vitamin K is synthesized in the intestines of newborns, and since their intestinal flora are often underdeveloped at birth, there may not be enough Vitamin K synthesized. This can lead to hemorrhagic disease or navel bleeding in newborn babies. An intramuscular injection of Vitamin K at birth can help ward off such problems by supplying the newborn with the Vitamin K that he/she needs until the newborn is able to synthesize enough Vitamin K independently.

RESPIRATORY ACIDOSIS

Respiratory acidosis is a condition in which there is an increased retention of carbon dioxide by the lungs. This retention upsets the acid-base balance of the patient's blood and an increased level of dissolved carbon dioxide in the blood, in conjunction with a normal or elevated level of bicarbonate in the blood. The increased dissolved carbon dioxide in the blood is often due to hypoventilation from respiratory problems, including pneumonia, asthma, and bronchitis.

METABOLIC ACIDOSIS

Metabolic acidosis is an increase in the acidity of blood plasma due to a high formation of organic acids in the body. These acids form at such a fast rate that is greater than the rate at which they break down. This rate discrepancy is what leads to metabolic acidosis. There are several possible causes of metabolic acidosis: Lowered blood pH; renal failure, causing a reduction in the amount of acid excreted by the kidneys; uncontrolled diabetes, which leads to an increased production of ketone bodies (such as acetoacetic acid and other acids); and using diuretics, which increase the amount of bicarbonate that is excreted in the urine.

STANDARD BICARBONATE AND TOTAL CO_2

Standard Bicarbonate: Standard bicarbonate is defined as the concentration of bicarbonate in the blood. In order to determine standard bicarbonate, the carbon gas that is dissolved in the blood must be equilibrated to 40 mm Hg, and the blood sample must be fully oxygenated at 37 degrees Celsius.

Total CO_2: Total CO_2 (carbon dioxide) of blood plasma is defined as the sum of the bicarbonate and the dissolved carbon dioxide present in the plasma. This is a measure of the concentration of the dissolved carbon dioxide, carbonic acid, carbonate, bicarbonate, and carbamino compounds present in the plasma. Bicarbonate makes up the greatest portion of the total carbon dioxide.

HENDERSON-HASSELBALCH EQUATION

The Henderson-Hasselbalch equation is pH = pk` + log ([salt]/[acid]). pk` is the acid dissociation constant (also written as pk_a). The equation describes how the pH of a solution can vary as the ratio of salt to acid (or the acidity) also varies. In terms of the medical laboratory, it can be used to determine the acid-base equilibrium of the blood.

TESTS FOR ACID-BASE BALANCE

Arterial blood gases are monitored to assess effectiveness of oxygenation, ventilation, and acid-base status, and to determine oxygen flow rates. Partial pressure of a gas is that exerted by each gas in a mixture of gases, proportional to its concentration, based on total atmospheric pressure of 760 mm Hg at sea level. Normal values include:

- Acidity/alkalinity (pH): 7.35-7.45.
- Partial pressure of carbon dioxide ($PaCO_2$): 35-45 mm Hg.
- Partial pressure of oxygen (PaO_2): ≥80 mg Hg.
- Bicarbonate concentration (HCO_3): 22-26 mEq/L.
- Oxygen saturation (SaO_2): ≥95%.

The relationship between these elements indicates respiratory and metabolic status. Decreased bicarbonate and PaO2 occur with metabolic acidosis and respiratory alkalosis. Increased bicarbonate and PaO2 occur with metabolic alkalosis and respiratory acidosis.

PHARMACOKINETICS

Pharmacokinetics include the route of administration, the absorption, the dosage, the frequency of administration, the distribution, and the serum levels achieved over time. The drug's rate of clearance (elimination) and doses needed to ensure therapeutic benefit must be considered. Most drugs are cleared through the kidneys, with water-soluble compounds excreted more readily than protein-soluble compounds. Volume of distribution (IV drug dose divided by plasma concentration) determines the rate at which the drug passes into tissue. Drug distribution depends on the degree of protein binding and ion trapping that takes place. Effect-site equilibrium is the time between administration of a drug and clinical effect (the point at which the drug reaches the appropriate receptors) and must be considered when determining dose, time, and frequency of drugs. The bioavailability of drugs may vary, depending upon the degree of metabolism that takes place before the drug reaches its site of action.

CONFIRMATORY TESTS AND TOXICOLOGICAL TESTS

Screening tests determine if classes of drugs (such as opioids) are present. **Confirmatory tests** determine if a false negative or positive has occurred and identifies specific drugs. **Toxicological tests** assess the presence or level of drugs or other substances in blood, urine, hair, or saliva and therapeutic drug monitoring (TDM).

Drug abuse	"Tox screen" tests for multiple drugs, other screening panels.
Antiepileptics (AEDs) & metabolites	AED/TDM (usually trough). With adverse effects, test when symptoms occur (most often 4-6 hours after administration).
Cardioactive drugs & metabolites	Digoxin test to monitor therapeutic levels and diagnose toxicity.
Immunosuppressives	TDM (trough levels) for cyclosporine, tacrolimus, sirolimus, and other drugs.

PRINCIPLES OF THERAPEUTIC DRUG MONITORING

Plasma drug levels are used for **therapeutic drug monitoring** because, although plasma is often not the site of action, plasma levels correlate well with therapeutic and toxic responses to most drugs. The therapeutic range of a drug is that between the minimum effective concentration (level at which there is no therapeutic benefit) and the toxic concentration (level at which toxic effects occur). To achieve drug plateau (steady state), the drug half-life (time needed to decrease drug concentration by 50%) must be considered. Most drugs reach plateau with administration equal to 4 half-lives and completely eliminate a drug in 5 half-lives. Because drug levels fluctuate, peak (highest drug concentration) and trough (lowest drug concentration) levels may be monitored. Samples for trough levels are taken immediately prior to administration of another dose while peak samples are taken at various times, depending on the average peak time of the specific drug, which may vary from 30 minutes to about 2 hours after administration.

BARBITURATES

Barbiturates are a class of drug that acts as a depressant or a body sedative. These drugs depress the activity of the nervous system, including parts of the brain. Barbiturates depress the functions of all body tissues to some extent. Barbiturates lower blood pressure and respiratory rate. Small doses of barbiturates induce sleepiness and drowsiness, while high doses act as anesthetics, and

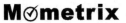

overdoses can even cause coma and death. The barbiturates are differentiated according to their activity level: Long- acting, intermediate-acting, short-acting, and very short-acting barbiturates. The long-acting barbiturates have increased therapeutic duration when compared to the shorter acting barbiturates. Long-acting barbiturates require higher doses to be toxic. Some examples of barbiturates include: Phenobarbital (long- acting), amobarbital (intermediate-acting), pentobarbital (short- acting), and thiopental sodium (very short-acting).

PHARMACODYNAMICS

Pharmacodynamics relates to biological effects (therapeutic or adverse) of drug administration over time. Drug transport, absorption, means of elimination, and half-life must all be considered when determining effects. Responses may include continuous responses, such as blood pressure variations, or dichotomous response in which an event either occurs or does not (such as death). Information from pharmacodynamics provides feedback to modify medication dosage (pharmacokinetics). Drugs provide biological effects primarily by interacting with receptor sites (specific protein molecules) in the cell membrane. Receptors include voltage-sensitive ion channels (sodium, chloride, potassium, and calcium channels), ligand-gated ion channels, and transmembrane receptors. Agonist drugs exert effects after binding with a receptor while antagonist drugs bind with a receptor but have no effects, so they can block agonists from binding. The total number of receptors may vary, upregulating or downregulating in response to stimuli (such as drug administration). Dose-response curves show the relationship between the amount of drug given and the resultant plasma concentration and biological effects.

TOXICOLOGICAL TESTS

Screening tests determine if classes of drugs (such as opioids) are present. **Confirmatory tests** determine if a false negative or positive has occurred and identifies specific drugs. **Toxicological tests** assess the presence or level of drugs or other substances in blood, urine, hair, or saliva and therapeutic drug monitoring (TDM).

Antidepressants	Antidepressant drug profile (urine) shows presence of multiple antidepressants. TDM used for specific drugs.
Antibiotics	Aminoglycoside test used to monitor drug levels 6-144 hours after dose. Specific TDM for different antibiotics.
Beta blockers	BB panel tests for multiple drugs. Hypoglycemia is common with BB toxicity.
Calcium channel blockers	TDM. With toxicity, multiple other tests (glucose, electrolytes, blood gases, ECG) are needed. Hyperglycemia is common with CCB toxicity.

ENZYME-MULTIPLIED IMMUNOASSAY TECHNIQUE (EMIT)

The enzyme-multiplied immunoassay technique is used to determine the concentration of a particular drug in a serum sample by using an enzyme label. First, an antibody that is specific to the drug in question is added to the sample. Secondly, a coenzyme and a substrate for the enzyme label are then added to the serum sample. Finally, the free labeled antigen (the enzyme labeled drug) is added to the serum sample. The enzyme labeled drug that has been added to the serum then competes with the particular drug in question that is already present in the serum sample for binding sites on the antibody that had been added. When the enzyme labeled drug binds to the antibody, decreased enzyme activity is exhibited, resulting in the free enzyme labeled drug being the only thing that can react with the substrate and the coenzyme. Enzyme activity is measured at 340 nm, and it is directly proportional to the amount of the particular drug in the serum. The higher the concentration of the particular drug in the serum, the higher the amount of enzyme activity.

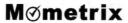

REINSCH'S TEST

The Reinsch's Test is a laboratory test used to determine the presence of heavy metals in a sample, often urine. In this particular test, the urine sample is dissolved in a solution of hydrochloric acid (HCl). After the urine is dissolved, a strip of copper is placed into the solution. If a heavy metal is present, the copper strip will develop a colored coating. A silver coating may indicate the presence of mercury, while a blackish/blue color (or another dark color) may indicate the presence of another heavy metal, such as antimony, arsenic, bismuth, selenium, or thallium. The test is a rapid one, and is good for a quick, initial screening. However, the findings of this test should be confirmed with other laboratory techniques.

TRINDER REACTION

The Trinder Reaction is used most often to determine the presence of salicylate in the urine. A solution containing ferric chloride is added to the urine sample in question. An iron complex will form between the ferric chloride and the salicylate, if salicylate is present. This reaction will turn the solution a purple color. The test is very rapid, and this is one of its positive points. However, the test has the possibility for false positive results as well. A purple color will also be produced if any enol or phenol is present in the urine, as well as if the patient has an elevated urine bilirubin level of 1 mg/dL or greater.

PRINCIPLES OF FETAL WELLNESS TESTS

Lecithin/sphingomyelin (L/S) ratio: The ratio of the phospholipids lecithin and sphingomyelin (two components of surfactant) changes during pregnancy with L/S ratio at 0.5:1 early in pregnancy, 1:1 at 30-32 weeks, and 2:1 at 35 weeks. This test is not accurate if the amniotic fluid contains blood or meconium. **Alpha-fetoprotein (AFT)** is a protein produced by the yolk sac for the first 6 weeks of gestation and then by the fetal liver. Cutoff levels have been established for each week of gestation, with peak levels at about week 15. The test is used primarily to detect neural tube defects (NTDs), which develop in the first trimester. AFT can be measured in amniotic fluid or maternal serum. **Delta 450** is an amniotic bilirubin scan, usually done only with fetal transfusion because it requires amniocentesis. **Fibronectin** (an adhesive glycoprotein that adheres fetal membrane to placenta) is measured in vaginal secretions and is present early in pregnancy and near term (after week 35). Earlier detection may indicate preterm labor.

MINERALS OF THE BODY AND MINERAL METABOLISM

Minerals are essential to the body and include major essential minerals for which >100 mg/dL is required (calcium, chloride, fluoride, magnesium, phosphorous, potassium, sodium, and sulphur); trace elements for which <100 mg/dL is required (copper, iodine, iron, manganese, molybdenum, selenium, and zinc); and multiple other elements that the body uses in ways that are not completely understood (nickel, bromide, barium). Absorption of minerals is complex and may occur anywhere in the GI tract, but most occurs in the small intestine in the duodenum and jejunum. For example, calcium absorption (small intestine) is stimulated by increased release of parathormone and dependent on vitamin D. Transporters, such as transferrin, may be needed to carry the mineral to cells. Absorption increases when body stores are low. Some minerals are co-transported with other substances, such as sodium with amino acids or glucose. Disorders occur when mineral levels are too high or too low.

METABOLISM OF PURINES, FORMATION OF URIC ACID, AND TESTS FOR GOUT

Gout (metabolic arthritis) is a group of conditions associated with a defect of purine metabolism, resulting in hyperuricemia with oversecretion of uric acid, decreased excretion of uric acid, or a combination. Purine is ingested in food, especially meats. Increased uric acid levels can cause monosodium urate crystal depositions in the joints, resulting in severe articular and periarticular inflammation. With chronic gout, sodium urate crystals, called tophi, accumulate in peripheral body areas, such as the great toe (75%), ankle, knee, hands, and ears. Assessment is through uric acid levels:

Normal values: Male 4.4 to 7.6 mg/dL, Female 2.3 to 6.6 mg/dL.

Crystals may begin to form with levels >7. Testing is carried out on 1 mL serum collected in a red- or tiger-capped or heparinized green-capped tube. If the patient is receiving rasburicase, the specimen must be collected in a pre-chilled heparinized green-capped tube and transported in ice slurry. Analysis is done with spectrophotometry. A joint fluid test with microscopic analysis may also be carried out with aspirated synovial fluid.

PROBLEMS MAY OCCUR WHEN PERFORMING ELECTROPHORESIS

Very slow migration: voltage too low; ionic charge too low; molecular weight too high; ionic strength too high;

No migration: incorrect pH buffer; apparatus not connected to electrical outlet; electrodes connected improperly

Holes in the staining pattern: concentration of analyte is too high

Precipitation of the sample in the support media: excessive heating; pH too high or too low

REFERENCE RANGES

1. Total calcium: 8.7 to 10.2 mg/dL
2. Magnesium: 1.6 to 2.4 mg/dL
3. Phosphorus: 2.7 to 4.5 mg/dL
4. Bilirubin: 0.2 to 1.0 mg/dL
5. Urobilinogen: 0.1 to 1.0 mg/dL every 2 hours
6. Fasting glucose: 70 to 115 mg/dL
7. BUN (blood urea nitrogen): 7 to 18 mg/dL
8. Uric acid: 3.5 to 7.2 mg/dL
9. Creatinine: 0.7 to 1.2 mg/dL
10. total cholesterol: 140-270 mg/dL (male); 140-242 mg/dL (female)
11. triglycerides: 50-321 mg/dL (male); 52-262 (female)
12. HDL: 28-75 mg/dL (male); 33-92 mg/dL (female)
13. LDL: 70-186 (male); 71-206 mg/dL (female)
14. Apo-A: 120-160 mg/dL
15. Apo-B: less than 120 mg/dL
16. Lp(a): less than 30 mg/dL

FRIEDEWALD FORMULA AND CALCULATING THE LDL OF A MAN WITH TOTAL CHOLESTEROL = 160 MG/DL; HDL = 50 MG/DL; TRIGLYCERIDES = 120

The Friedewald formula is a means of calculating LDL cholesterol level when the total cholesterol, HDL cholesterol, and triglyceride levels are known. The formula is as follows: LDL cholesterol = total cholesterol – [HDL cholesterol + triglycerides/5]. The Friedewald formula cannot be used when the triglyceride level exceeds 400 mg/dL.

SUBSTRATE CONCENTRATION EFFECT ON THE RATE OF AN ENZYME REACTION

It is typical for substrate concentration to be directly proportional to the rate of an enzyme reaction. It is possible, however, for a maximum limit of reaction to be reached. This occurs when there is so much substrate present that substrate binds to all of the available enzymes. Of course, the formation of more products will enable the creation of more enzymes.

RELATION OF INHIBITOR TO ENZYMES

Inhibitor: any substance that is catalyzed by an enzyme and interferes with reaction; may be reversible or irreversible

RELATION OF COMPETITIVE INHIBITOR TO ENZYMES

Competitive inhibitor: any substance that attempts to bind to an enzyme's active site, preventing the substrate from binding there; this is reversible inhibition

RELATION OF NONCOMPETITIVE INHIBITOR TO ENZYMES

Noncompetitive inhibitor: a substance that attempts to bind to the enzyme at a place other than the active site; inhibition can be reversible or irreversible

SYMPTOMS OF A TOXIC OVERDOSE

1. Valproic acid: weight gain, nausea, pancreatitis, hallucinations, and lethargy
2. lithium: lethargy, difficulty with speech, muscle weakness, apathy, and, in extreme doses, seizures and coma
3. Tricyclic antidepressants: constipation, seizures, drowsiness, memory loss, blurred vision, and, in extreme doses, seizures, unconsciousness, and cardiac arrhythmia
4. Cyclosporine: renal tubular and glomerular dysfunction
5. Theophylline: diarrhea, nausea, vomiting, and, at extreme doses, seizures and cardiac arrhythmia
6. Digoxin: vomiting, vision problems, premature ventricular contractions, and nausea

ACID-BASE BUFFER SYSTEMS

1. Phosphate buffer system: a system that uses the HPO_4^{-2} and $H_2PO_4^-$ ions in body cells to diminish changes in pH in the cells of the body
2. Bicarbonate buffer system: a system that uses HCO_3^- and H_2CO_3 in the blood to diminish changes in pH in the blood
3. Hemoglobin buffer system: a system that uses a hemoglobin in plasma and red blood cells to diminish changes in pH in the blood
4. Protein buffer system: a system that uses plasma proteins to diminish changes in pH in the blood

EFFECTS OF BREATHING ON BLOOD pH

The rate of breathing has a direct effect on the balance between acids and bases in the blood. When an individual breathes extremely slowly, excess carbon dioxide will accumulate in the lungs and in the blood. The results will be a reduced pH, because of the increase in carbonic acid. When an individual breathes rapidly, the accelerated evacuation of carbon dioxide will result in an increase of bicarbonate ions in the blood, which in turn causes the pH of the blood to increase.

TYPES OF HYPONATREMIA

Individuals suffering from hyponatremia have a sodium level less than 136 mEq/L. Hyponatremia comes in two varieties: depletional and dilutional. Depletional hyponatremia is caused by low water volume, which may be the result of diuretics, excessive sweating, diarrhea, or vomiting. Dilutional hyponatremia, on the other hand, is caused by high water volume, which may be the result of congestive heart failure, over consumption of water, hypothyroidism, or cirrhosis. Individuals suffering from hyponatremia will complain of nausea, lethargy, and headaches. In severe cases, seizure or coma may occur.

ANION GAP

The anion gap differentiates between metabolic acidosis conditions, and indicates the relative electro-neutrality of body fluids. The formula for the anion gap is as follows: (sodium concentration + potassium concentration) – (chloride concentration + bicarbonate concentration). The normal range is between 10 and 20 mmol/L. If the level is lower than normal, this may be because of the presence of paraproteins resulting from multiple myeloma or hypoalbuminemia. If levels are higher than normal, this is likely the result of renal failure, lactic acidosis, ketoacidosis, or the consumption of antibiotics, methanol, or salicylate.

STRUCTURE OF A PROTEIN

Proteins, otherwise known as polypeptides, are made up of amino acid polymers joined together by covalent bonds. The primary structure of a protein is simply the carbon and all groups directly connected to carbon. The secondary structure of a protein includes the beta sheets, alpha helixes, and coils that join together. The tertiary structure of a protein is the protein's folding, the result of interactions between ionized side chains. The quaternary structure of a protein is all the peptide chains bound together. The N-terminal end of a protein has a free amino group, while the C-terminal end has a free carboxyl group.

SIMPLE PROTEINS VS. CONJUGATED PROTEINS

Simple proteins consist only of amino acids, and may be either globular or fibrous. Albumin is an example of a globular protein, while collagen is an example of a fibrous protein. A conjugated protein, meanwhile, is one that contains a prosthetic, nonprotein group. Nucleoproteins, glycoproteins, lipoproteins, metalloproteins are all examples of conjugated proteins. A nucleoprotein is attached to a nucleic acid; a glycoprotein is attached to a carbohydrate; a lipoprotein is attached to lipids; a metalloprotein is attached to a metal group.

HYPERLIPOPROTEINEMIAS

1. Type I: serum appearance features a creamy layer; on a cholesterol test, HDL level is normal and LDL level is high; triglyceride test values are normal
2. Type IIa: serum appearance is clear; HDL level is normal and LDL level is extremely high; triglyceride values are normal
3. Type IIb: serum appears cloudy or clear; high VLDL and LDL; triglycerides are high
4. Type III: serum is cloudy with a creamy layer on top; total cholesterol is higher than normal; triglycerides are higher than normal
5. Type IV: serum appears hazy or cloudy; cholesterol levels are normal; triglycerides are elevated
6. Type V: serum appears cloudy or creamy; cholesterol is very high; triglycerides are very high

ACCEPTED DESIRABLE AND HIGH-RISK VALUES

1. Total cholesterol: desirable: less than 200 mg/dL; high risk: more than 240 mg/dL; borderline: 200-239 mg/dL
2. HDL cholesterol: desirable: more than 60 mg/dL; high risk: less than 35 mg/dL

3. LDL cholesterol: desirable values: less than 130 mg/dL; high risk: more than 160 mg/dL; borderline: 130-159 mg/dL
4. Triglycerides: desirable: less than 250 mg/dL; high risk: more than 400 mg/dL; borderline: 130-159 mg/dL

LIPOPROTEINS AND THEIR COMPOSITION

1. Chylomicrons: the lightest lipoprotein, absorbed by the intestine; transports triglycerides after a meal; composed of 90% triglycerides, and 5% cholesterol, 3% phospholipids, and 2% protein
2. Very low density lipoproteins (VLDL): carries fats and triglycerides; produced by the liver and decomposed by muscle and adipose tissue; composed of 60% triglycerides, 20% cholesterol, 14% phospholipids, and 2% protein
3. Low density lipoproteins (LDL): carries bad cholesterol; composed of 40% cholesterol, 22% phospholipids, 20% triglycerides, and 18% protein
4. High density lipoproteins (HDL): carries good cholesterol; composed of 44% protein, 26% phospholipids, 25% cholesterol, and 5% triglycerides

PEPTIDES AND STEROIDS

Peptides are hormones that initiate chemical responses in the body by means of their reactions to receptors on cell membranes. Unlike steroids, peptide hormones do not require a carrier protein. Some common examples of peptide hormones are insulin, prolactin, parathyroid hormone, thyroid stimulating hormone, and luteinizing hormone. Steroids must be accompanied by a carrier protein, and are only produced by the gonads, adrenal glands, and placenta when they are needed. Testosterone, cortisol, progesterone, and estrogen are all common examples of steroid hormones.

QUALITATIVE AND QUANTITATIVE TEST METHODS FOR DETERMINING THE PRESENCE OF FECAL FAT

There are both qualitative and quantitative means of identifying malabsorbed fat in feces. The quantitative method involves collecting stool samples over a period of 72 hours, mixing the samples, and analyzing a small sample. The level of fats in the sample can be measured through the process known as saponification. The qualitative method of measuring fecal fat is to take a random stool sample and combine it with a fat-soluble stain on a microscope slide. Sudan III, Sudan IV, Nile Blue, and Oil Red O are all used for this purpose. Malabsorbed fecal fat will present as reddish orange oil bubbles.

LACTOSE TOLERANCE TEST

The ability of the digestive system to process lactose can be measured with the lactose tolerance test. In a normal human, the enzyme lactase divides lactose into two components, galactose and glucose. For this reason, in a normal person blood glucose level will rise after the consumption of lactose. However, individuals unable to process lactose will not experience an increase in blood glucose level. The lactose tolerance test is performed as follows: the individual receives a preliminary blood draw, then drinks a liquid with 50 g of lactose. Glucose levels of the blood are checked at regular intervals; if the blood glucose levels increase by 30 mg/dL or more, lactose is being processed properly.

REFERENCE RANGES VARIOUS HORMONES

1. Growth hormone: less than 10 ng/mL (females); less than 2 ng/dL (males); anterior pituitary gland
2. Prolactin: 5 to 40 ng/mL (females); 0 to 20 ng/mL (males); anterior pituitary gland

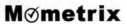

3. Aldosterone: 5-30 pg/dL (females); 6-22 pg/dL (males); adrenal glands
4. Cortisol: 5 to 23 µg/mL (morning); 3-16 µg/mL (evening); adrenal glands

URINALYSIS TERMINOLOGY

Prerenal	Classification of kidney disorders caused by problems outside of (before) the kidney, such as inadequate blood flow.
Suprapubic	Above the pubic bone, often the place where suprapubic catheters are placed, especially in males requiring long-term catheterization.
Glycosuria	Presence of glucose in the urine.
Renal threshold	The concentration at which the kidneys begin to remove a substance from the blood and into the urine.
Ascites	Accumulation of serous fluid in the abdominal cavity.
Tamm-Horsfall protein	AKA uromodulin, the most common protein found in normal urine.
Myoglobin	Protein found in muscle tissue.
Amniocentesis	Transabdominal sampling of amniotic fluid from the amniotic sac for prenatal diagnoses of chromosomal disorders and infections.
Pass-through	Duration of time that a drug needs to pass-through the liver and/or kidney.
Osmolality	Concentration of a substance (blood/urine).
Xanthochromic	Yellow-colored, usually in reference to cerebrospinal fluid that has the appearance of urine.

Hematology

HEMATOLOGY TERMINOLOGY

Nucleated RBC (NRBC)	Immature red blood cell that contain a nucleus, abnormal when found in peripheral blood.
Hematocrit	Percentage of erythrocytes in whole blood.
Reticulocyte	Immature erythrocyte that shows a basophilic reticulum under vital staining.
Hematopoiesis	Formation and maturation of blood cells.
Differential	Different types of leukocytes by percentage (monocytes, lymphocytes, neutrophils, basophils, and eosinophils)
Plasma	Liquid portion of blood or lymph.
Leukemia	Malignancy of blood-forming organs with abnormal proliferation and development of leukocytes and precursors.
Buffy coat	In centrifuged blood, the layer of leukocytes above the packed red blood cells.
Hypertonic	A solution with greater osmotic pressure than the solution to which it is compared.
Hypotonic	A solution with lower osmotic pressure than the solution to which it is compared.
Sodium citrate	Crystalline compound used as an anticoagulant and retains coagulation factors

THROMBOCYTES AND ERYTHROCYTES

Thrombocyte: Thrombocyte is another word for platelet. A platelet is a type of blood cell that is small in size, irregular in its shape, and colorless. Platelets play an important role in the clotting and coagulation of blood, and they can also aid in helping to repair injured blood vessels. Platelets are produced by the bone marrow and are stored in the spleen.

Erythrocyte: A erythrocyte is a red blood cell (RBC). Red blood cells are cells that carry oxygen from the lungs to the rest of the body's tissues. These cells are red because of the hemoglobin that they contain. RBCs are produced by the bone marrow, especially of the long bones, and stored in the spleen.

GRANULOCYTES

Granulocyte: A granulocyte is a type of white blood cell that has granules in its cytoplasm. There are three types of granulocytes: basophils, eosinophils, and neutrophils. Approximately 75% of all white blood cells are granulocytes.

LYMPHOCYTES

Lymphocyte: Lymphocytes are a special type of white blood cell that play an important role in the immune system. B cells and T cells are the two types of lymphocytes.

MONOCYTES

Monocyte: A monocyte is another type of white blood cell. These cells are characterized by a well-defined nucleus. They play an important role in the body's immune response to pathogens. These cells are also produced in the bone marrow.

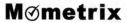

ERYTHROPOIETINS

Erythropoietin is a particular hormone that is responsible in increasing the production of red blood cells in the body. Erythropoietin is a glycoprotein hormone, or a protein with a sugar attached to it. Erythropoietin is released when there is a lower level of oxygen in the body's tissues, implying a reduced amount of red blood cells (anemia), so the erythropoietin helps replenish these red blood cells to increase oxygen levels in the body. Erythropoietin is produced mainly in the kidneys, but there is evidence that it may also be produced, in part, by the liver. Dialysis patients or those undergoing chemotherapy) may not be able to produce enough erythropoietin on their own, so they can take a synthetic form of erythropoietin to aid in the replenishment of red blood cells to prevent severe anemia, or receive packed cell transfusions.

TYPES OF GRANULOCYTES

These three types of granulocytes are distinguished by their ability to be stained with various types of stains in the laboratory. Basophils are stained black by basic stains, eosinophils are stained red by acid stains, and neutrophils are stained pale lilac by neutral pH stains. Basophils play an important role in allergies and allergic reactions, as well as in inflammation. Eosinophils play an important part in the defense against infection by parasites, and neutrophils take part in the defense against infection from microorganisms.

PHAGOCYTES AND IMMUNOCYTES

A phagocyte is a type of leukocyte (white blood cell) that participates in phagocytosis (cell digestion). Phagocytes use enzymes to help digest pieces of other cells, cell debris, waste materials, foreign bodies, or harmful organisms that can be found in the body's tissues and bloodstream. Granulocytes (eosinophils, basophils, and neutrophils) and monocytes (macrophages) are all types of phagocytes. An immunocyte is also a type of leukocyte that is found in the body's lymphatic system. Immunocytes produce antibodies to help fight viruses and other diseases. The lymphocytes (B-lymphocytes and T-lymphocytes) are types of immunocytes.

T-LYMPHOCYTES AND B-LYMPHOCYTES

T-lymphocytes are white blood cells responsible for the body's cell-mediated immune system response to a viral or bacterial infection. This response is accomplished through the antigens on specific T- lymphocytes that have the ability to destroy cells that have been infected by a virus, bacteria, other microbe, or cancerous cells. B-lymphocytes, on the other hand, are a type of lymphocyte that combats infection or viruses through the use of antibodies, called humoral immunity. In humoral immunity, B-lymphocytes secrete specific antibodies into the blood plasma, and these antibodies attach themselves to specific antigens. Antigens can be located on viruses, bacteria, or other microbes. The binding of the antibodies to the antigens then signals to the body that these are the cells that should be lyzed or subjected to phagocytosis.

HOWELL-JOLLY BODIES, HEINZ BODIES, AND SCHISTOCYTES

Howell-Jolly bodies consist of DNA remnants. They are found as clusters in red blood cells where the division of the cell's nucleus was incomplete. Howell-Jolly bodies are often found in patients with a missing or damaged spleen. Heinz bodies are made up of denatured hemoglobin. They are seen as spots in red blood cells. Schistocytes are red blood cell pieces or fragments, often with abnormal shapes. They are usually indicative of hemolysis or damage to small blood vessels.

LEUKEMOID REACTION

A leukemoid reaction is a case of leukocytosis (an elevated white blood cell count) in healthy bone marrow that is similar to leukemia, but is caused by infection, trauma, high stress, hemorrhage, or unknown causes. Patients with tuberculosis, whooping cough, or other diseases that produce a cytokine storm may show leukemoid reactions. A white blood cell count over 25 to 30 x 10^9/L, with many mature neutrophils in the differential, and an elevated LAP are indicative of a leukemoid reaction. A patient with leukemia would have many immature neutrophils in the smear, instead. A leukemoid reaction is synonymous with a transient myoproliferative reaction.

RED BLOOD CELL INDICES

1. Mean corpuscular volume (MCV): calculated as hematocrit divided by red blood cell count; indicates average volume of individual red blood cells; normal range between 80 and 95 femtoliters (fL); a low MCV is sometimes the result of anemia or liver disease
2. Mean corpuscular hemoglobin (MCH): calculated as hemoglobin divided by red blood cell count; indicates average weight of hemoglobin in each red blood cell; normal range is 26 to 34 picograms; a low MCH is sometimes the result of microcytic anemia, while a high MCH is sometimes the result of macrocytic anemia
3. Mean corpuscular hemoglobin concentration (MCHC): calculated as hemoglobin concentration divided by hematocrit, and multiplied by 100; indicates average concentration of hemoglobin in grams per deciliter (g/dL) of red blood cells; normal range is 32 to 36%; low levels may be the result of thalassemia or anemia, while high levels may indicate spherocytosis
4. Hematocrit (HCT): the volume of packed red blood cells; the ratio of red blood cells in whole blood; normal range is 40 to 52%

MOLECULAR CONTENT HEMOGLOBIN, BART'S HEMOGLOBIN, METHEMOGLOBIN, AND CARBOXYHEMOGLOBIN

Hemoglobin is made up of four globin chains (two alpha and two beta, in a human adult) and four heme molecules. Bart's hemoglobin is made up of four globin chains as well, but they are all gamma chains. Methemoglobin consists of hemoglobin that has had the iron in the heme groups oxidized from its ferrous form to its ferric form. Carboxyhemoglobin is hemoglobin that has a carboxy (CO) group attached to the iron in the heme molecules.

FUNCTION OF BONE MARROW

The process of production and differentiation of blood cells is known as hematopoiesis. The process works as follows: bone marrow produces stem cells, which in turn differentiate into colony forming units and then, subsequently, into monocytes, granulocytes, erythrocytes, thrombocytes, T-lymphocytes, and B-lymphocytes. Bone marrow also produces progenitor cells and precursor cells. Precursor cells develop into blasts, while progenitor cells differentiate into a single cell line, either granulocyte, thrombocyte, or erythrocyte.

MATURATION SERIES OF ERYTHROCYTES AND ERYTHROCYTE PRODUCTION AND DESTRUCTION

Erythrocyte maturation series: All blood cells develop from hematocytoblast stem cells:

- College of American Pathologists: Pronormoblast—basophilic normoblast (erythroblast)—polychromatophilic normoblast—orthochromic normoblast—reticulocyte—erythrocyte.
- American Society for Clinical Pathologists: Rubriblast—prorubricyte—rubricyte—metarubricyte—reticulocyte—erythrocyte.

The first 4 stages of both classification systems contain a nucleus, which gets smaller and disappears from reticulocytes or mature erythrocytes. The first 3 stages are found in the bone marrow but the immature cells of stage 4 and stage 5 (reticulocytes) may enter the peripheral blood when production is high. **Erythrocyte production (erythropoiesis) and destruction**: Kidneys produce erythropoietin in response to decreased oxygen level in the blood, stimulating the bone marrow to produce erythrocytes. The lifespan of an erythrocyte is about 120 days with 2 to 3 million circulating in an average adult. Production falls when oxygen levels rise. Aging erythrocytes are removed in the spleen and liver by macrophages. Some component parts are reused: Iron returns to the bone marrow, heme is broken down into bilirubin for excretion, and globin is reused or reduced to amino acids.

MATURATION SERIES OF GRANULOCYTES AND AGRANULOCYTES

Granulocytes (neutrophils, eosinophils, basophils) with lobed nuclei and granules	Agranulocytes (monocytes, lymphocytes) with single-lobe nuclei and no granules
Myeloid progenitor	**Monocyte:** Myeloid progenitor Monoblast (12-20 µm) with large oval nucleus and lymphoid dendritic cells Promonocyte (from monoblast) Monocyte Macrophage and myeloid dendritic cell.
Myeloblast (10-20 µm): oval nucleus with no granules evident in cytoplasm.	**Lymphocyte:** Common lymphoid progenitor Lymphoblast (10-20 µm) with large round nucleus. Prolymphocyte Small lymphocyte and natural killer cell B and T lymphoctyes (from small lymphocyte)
Promyelocyte (10-20 µm): Granules in cytoplasm.	
Myelocyte (10-18 µm): Large oval nucleus. Primary granules evident but secondary more prevalent.	
Metamyelocyte (10-18 µm): Kidney-shaped nucleus with primary and secondary (most prevalent) granules.	
Band: U-shaped nucleus, secondary or neutrophilic or basophils granules most common.	
Segmented cells (14 µm): 2-5 joined lobes.	

THROMBOCYTE (PLATELET) MATURATION SERIES AND BLOOD SMEAR FOR PLATELETS

The **thrombocyte maturation series** includes:

- Hemocytoblast (able to produce all cell types)
- Myeloid stem cells
- Megakaryoblast (21-50 µm) with irregular-shaped nucleus.
- Promegakaryocyte (20-80 µm) with 2-4 small nucleoli.

- Megakaryocyte (≤100 μm) with multi-lobed nucleus.
- Thrombocyte

<u>Count increased</u> in polycythemia vera, RA, acute infections, anemias, cirrhosis, chronic leukemia, splenectomy, TB, ulcerative colitis, and trauma. <u>Count decreased</u> in aplastic anemia, megaloblastic anemia, iron-deficiency anemia, idiopathic thrombocytopenia, severe hemorrhage, bone marrow replacement, radiation, multiple infections, lymphoma, aplastic anemia.

Blood smear for platelets may be carried out if the automated blood count shows an abnormally high or low. For the smear, a slide is treated with a stain and a drop of blood spread thinly across the slide. A microscopic examination or digital analyzer may be used to analyze the smear and determine the size and shape of the platelets. For example, if the platelets are exceptionally large ("giant") (the size of RBCs), this may be an indication of myeloproliferative neoplasm or immune thrombocytopenic purpura. A blood smear can also help to differentiate clumps of platelets from enlarged platelets.

T-CELL SUBSETS FUNCTIONS

1. T-helper cell: takes information about antigens from macrophages and monocytes and delivers that information to other cells; identified by cluster differentiation four-membrane proteins
2. T-suppressor cell: manages response of immune system; divided into three types: inducer, mediator, and effector; identified by the presence of cluster differentiation eight (CD8) membrane proteins
3. Cytotoxic T cell: contributes to the rejection of organs and the promotion of viral infections
4. T memory cell: over a long period of time, these cells respond to previously-introduced antigens

CYTOGENETIC ABNORMALITIES ASSOCIATED WITH HEMATOLOGIC NEOPLASMS

Abnormalities associated with hematologic neoplasms include:

- Auer bodies: Needle-like projections of crystalized granules in cytoplasm of myeloblasts and progranulocytes with some types of leukemia.
- Hypo-segmentation of neutrophils: <3 nuclear lobes, sometimes in odd shapes, indicate abnormal cell development.
- Smudge cells (basket cells): Cell remnants (especially lymphocytic) without nucleus or cytoplasmic membrane with leukemias, such as CLL.
- Abnormal cell count, increased or decreased.
- Abnormal cell size, small or enlarged.
- Hypo-granularity or hyper-granularity in granulocytes.
- Abnormal nuclei (folded, segmented, enlarged, abnormally shaped).
- Changes in cytoplasm (decreased or increased)
- Neutrophil abnormalities including neutrophilia, neutropenia, and or dysplastic neutrophils.
- Monocytosis with some types of leukemia.
- Presence of blast cells with bone marrow metastasis and leukemias.
- Plasma cells in blood with B-cell malignancy.
- Mast cells in blood with mast cell leukemia.

HEMOGLOBIN STRUCTURES

1. Fetal hemoglobin (Hb F): two gamma globin chains and two alpha globin chains
2. Hemoglobin Barts: four gamma globin chains and no alpha globin chains
3. Hemoglobin A: two alpha globin chains and two beta globin chains
4. Hemoglobin A_2: two alpha globin chains and two delta globin chains

RETICULOCYTES AND RETICULOCYTE COUNT

The last stage before maturity in the development of an erythrocyte is the appearance of the reticulocyte. These bodies do not contain a nucleus, although they do feature mitochondria and ribosomes. For adults, a normal range of reticulocytes is .5 to 1.5%, while for newborns the normal range is 2.5 to 6.5%. The reticulocyte count can be used as a gauge of bone marrow function and erythropoietic activity. These bodies can be viewed using a reticulocyte stain or a Wright stain.

TYPES OF ERYTHROCYTES

1. Macrocytes: erythrocytes with a mean corpuscular volume greater than 100 fL; indicates certain kinds of anemia
2. Echinocytes: erythrocytes with evenly-distributed spikes or bumps; may be caused by an elevated number of platelets
3. Keratocytes: erythrocytes with spiny extensions on the surface; possibly indicative of renal problems, ulcers, or liver disease
4. Acanthocytes: erythrocytes with irregularly-spaced spikes on the surface; possibly indicative of liver disease
5. Microcytes: erythrocytes with a mean corpuscular volume of less than 80 fL; may indicate certain kinds of anemia or thalassemia
6. Codocytes: erythrocytes consisting of a cell surrounded by successive concentric rings of hemoglobin, transparent material, and hemoglobin; may indicate liver disease, anemia, or another hemoglobinopathy
7. Spherocytes: small erythrocytes with no pale spot in the center; these also have an elevated mean corpuscular hemoglobin concentration; symptomatic of burns and hereditary spherocytosis
8. Schistocytes: erythrocytes fragments generated by movements through damaged blood vessels; symptomatic of burns
9. Dacrocytes: erythrocytes shaped like tears, and smaller than normal

ABNORMAL ERYTHROCYTE

1. Howell-Jolly bodies: fragments of DNA between 1 and 2 μm in size, and found in clusters among red blood cells; these bodies will test positive for the Feulgen stain, and will stain bluish-red to purple; typical of individuals with missing or damaged spleen, megaloblastic anemia, or sickle cell anemia
2. Pappenheimer bodies: clusters of iron granules found in an erythrocyte, typically at one end; turn dark blue or violet with Wright or Prussian Blue stain; caused by an aggregation of ribosomes, mitochondria, and iron fragments; characteristic of megaloblastic anemia, sideroblastic anemia, and thalassemia
3. Heinz bodies: denatured hemoglobin not usually included in an erythrocyte; 0.3 to 2.0 μm; identified with cresyl blue or crystal violet stains; typical of G6PD deficiency
4. Basophilic stippling: ribosomal RNA not usually included in an erythrocyte; inclusions may be fine or coarse, small or large; stains dark blue or purple; characteristic of lead poisoning, megaloblastic anemia, and thalassemia

DEVELOPMENT OF A PLATELET

1. Megakaryoblast: the first stage in platelet development; 20 to 50 μm; nucleus contains nucleoli; no visible chromatin; irregularly shaped cytoplasm with no granules; cytoplasm stains blue
2. Promegakaryocyte: slightly larger, 20 to 80 μm; contains double nucleus; cytoplasm as tags and granules; demarcating membrane system emerges
3. Megakaryocyte: between 30 and 100 μm; several nuclei; coarse chromatin; visible granules of blue and red
4. Metamegakaryocyte: largest cell in the human body; smaller nucleus to cytoplasm ratio; at this stage, platelets begin to detach from the demarcating membrane system

PLATELET COAGULATION GROUPS

1. Contact group: contains the coagulation factors XI, XII, high molecular weight kininogen, and prekallikrein; all of these factors are created in the liver and serve to activate fibrinolysis, intrinsic coagulation activation, and the activation of the complement system
2. Prothrombin group: contains coagulation factors II, VII, IX, and X; these factors are produced in the liver and require vitamin K; anticoagulation therapies and antibiotics may decrease the activity of these coagulation factors
3. Fibrinogen group: contains coagulation factors I, V, VIII, and XIII; these factors do not require vitamin K, and, with the exception of factor VIII, are located in platelets; these factors are substrates for the fibrinolytic enzyme plasmin

FIBRINOLYSIS AND COAGULATION INHIBITORS AND EFFECT OF HEPARIN

1. Alpha 2-antiplasmin: inhibits fibrinolysis; not affected by heparin
2. Alpha 1-antitrypsin: alters coagulation factor XI; not affected by heparin
3. Alpha 2-macroglobulin: alters the function and development of plasmin; not affected by heparin
4. Antithrombin III: obstructs the function of factors IX, X, XI, XII, plasmin, and kallikrein; made more effective by heparin
5. C1 inactivator: obstructs the function of factors XI, XII, and plasmin; not affected by heparin

USING HEMOCYTOMETER TO DETERMINE THE CONCENTRATION OF PARTICULAR CELLS IN A SAMPLE

Use a Neubauer-ruled hemocytometer to manually count blood cells or other microscopic particles in blood. The hemocytometer is a glass microscope slide with rectangular indentations that create a chamber with a depth of 0.1 mm. This chamber is scored with a series of perpendicular lines that form a grid (fields). Dilute a blood sample and pipette 10 microliters inside the chamber. Cover it with a glass coverslip. The diluted sample spreads across the chamber. Wait 10 minutes for cells to settle. Examine the chamber at 10x magnification under the microscope. Differentiate and count the cells in 9 large fields. Report the total WBC count per cubic millimeter as the (number of cells counted X10 X100)/9.

SCHILLING TEST

The Schilling test is used to determine if a deficiency in gastric intrinsic factor (IF) exists in a patient. In this test, the patient takes an oral radioactive isotope of Vitamin B_{12} labeled with cobalt, then completes a 24-hour urine collection. The isotope needs intrinsic factor in order to be adequately absorbed by the intestine, and then it should be excreted in the patient's urine. However, if the isotope collected in the urine is abnormally low (below 7%), not enough intrinsic factor is present. So the test is repeated, but this time with intrinsic factor added to the isotope, and

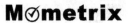

the amount of the isotope in the urine is determined again. If the amount of isotope in the second urine is at a normal level, then the patient is said to have a deficiency in the gastric intrinsic factor. This results in pernicious anemia, in which the patient has difficulty absorbing vitamin B_{12}. Pernicious anemia is common among vegans who have eaten no animal products for more than five years.

DISTINGUISHING ADULT HEMOGLOBIN (HB A) FROM FETAL HEMOGLOBIN (HB F)

One of the ways in which adult hemoglobin can be distinguished from fetal hemoglobin in the lab is through the Kleinhauer and Betke (KB) test. In this test, the red blood cells are treated with a citric acid-phosphate buffer solution that brings the pH down to 3.3. The red blood cells containing adult hemoglobin (Hb A) will become pale in color, while the red blood cells that contain fetal hemoglobin (Hb F) will remain stained. Alkaline electrophoresis can also help distinguish these two types of hemoglobin from each other. Because of its higher affinity for oxygen, the fetal hemoglobin will migrate more slowly during alkaline electrophoresis, as compared to the adult hemoglobin.

MEASURING HEMOGLOBIN IN THE LABORATORY

Hemoglobin can be measured in the laboratory using cyanide reagents. To measure hemoglobin, mix the blood sample with a solution containing potassium ferricyanide. The potassium ferricyanide oxidizes the iron found in the hemoglobin to its ferric state. Once its iron is oxidized, the hemoglobin is referred to as methemoglobin. Add potassium cyanide to the methemoglobin to form cyanmethemoglobin. Measure the cyanmethemoglobin using spectrophotometric techniques. The hemoglobin concentration present is proportional to the optical density of the cyanmethemoglobin formed in this reaction. The reagent used to measure hemoglobin used to be called Drabkin's reagent, but it is now called cyanmethemoglobin (HiCN) reagent.

OSMOTIC FRAGILITY TEST

The osmotic fragility test is based on the ability of a red blood cell to hold up when exposed to variances in salt concentration of a solution. Certain cells, such as spherocytes (spherical shaped red blood cells), will swell and eventually burst (hemolyze) as the salt concentration in the solution decreases. As the salt concentration decreases, more water will enter the red blood cell because of the principle of osmosis. If the cell has accepted the maximum amount of water that it can, but water is still trying to enter the red blood cell and the pressure inside the cell keeps increasing, the cell will burst, releasing hemoglobin (hemolysis). The reason that spherocytes are susceptible to hemolyzing in this test is because they have a low ratio of surface area to volume, as opposed to normal erythrocytes that are donut-shaped. Spherocytes are osmotically fragile -- not as resilient to pressure as are normally shaped erythrocytes.

COMPLETE BLOOD COUNT

A complete blood count, or CBC, consists of a white blood cell count, a red blood cell count, a platelet count, hemoglobin and mean cell volume, all of which are usually automated. A white blood cell differential is also performed manually on a smear if the doctor requests a diff. Hematocrit tubes are centrifuged to find the percentage of red cells by volume. Red blood cell indices are calculated using hemoglobin and hematocrit values with the red blood cell count. A complete blood cell count is performed to help diagnose a person with an infection, anemia, bleeding, leukemia, and some poisons. Pre-operative patients have a precautionary CBC before surgery. Complete blood cell counts can help a doctor check the progress of treatments for anemia, and the effectiveness of radiation and chemotherapy on cancers.

BONE MARROW ASPIRATION PROCEDURE

Bone marrow aspiration is usually done in the posterior superior (most common) or anterior superior iliac crest (or tibia for infants <1 year). Patients are placed in lateral decubitus or prone position, and adults receive local anesthesia and pediatric patients receive general anesthesia. Using aseptic technique, the procedure includes:

1. Infiltrating local anesthetic (10 mL/10% lidocaine).
2. Making small surgical incision.
3. Inserting aspiration needle through incision and into bone (turning back and forth to advance) until entering bone marrow cavity and then aspirating 0.3 mL bone marrow.
4. Immediately preparing slide or storing marrow in EDTA tube.
5. Removing needle, applying pressure, and applying dressing.

TOUCH PREPS FOR BONE MARROW BIOPSY AND ASPIRATION

Touch prep (to have 6 slides with morphological imprints of bone marrow biopsy):

1. Lay out 6 slides and place the marrow core on one.
2. Use a cover slide to roll the core across the first slide.
3. Use the second cover slide to roll the core across the second slide.
4. Use the third cover slide to roll the core across the third slide.
5. For aspirate, use smear technique (results in 1 slide), pull technique (2 slides), or lift technique (2 slides) (least effective method.)

INTERFERING FACTORS/SUBSTANCES IN HEMOGLOBIN MEASUREMENT

Tourniquet in place for >60 seconds	May increase levels up to 5%. Avoid extended use of tourniquet.
Rapid blood loss	Hgb may stay within normal parameters initially, so use other assessments.
Transfusion, recent	Hgb may remain unchanged initially, so be aware.
Cold agglutinins	May increase MCHC and decrease RBC count and hgb. Warm blood products, administer warm saline instead of plasma and recheck.
Positional change	Hgb may increase when upright and decrease when declining, so note position.
Hemolysis	Clotted or hemolyzed specimens should be rejected and specimen redrawn.
Lipids	May increase Hgb, MCV and MCHC. Administer warm saline instead of plasma and recheck and manually correct utilizing appropriate formula.
Copper deficiency	May decrease Hgb. Provide appropriate treatment.
RBC abnormalities	Some disorders, such as sickle cell disease, cause anemia and low Hgb. Treatment is usually provided to reach target Hgb.
Drugs	May increase or decrease Hgb. Note patient's medications.

WBC COUNT AND WBC DIFFERENTIAL

Automated methods of determining the **WBC count and differential** (and other cells) include hematology analyzers: Electrical impedance (blood cells pass through 2 electrodes and the impedance changes according to cell volume) and <u>flow cytometry</u> (uses lasers and reagents to pass blood cells through a laser beam to determine cell morphology). <u>Manual method</u>:

1. Gently mix blood with Turk diluent and wait 2 minutes for hemolysis to complete. 20× dilution is standard but high WBC counts may require up to 100× dilution.
2. Fill counting chamber by capillary and place on microscope stage.
3. Focus on one "W" marked area and count the cells in each square (cells blue with dark nucleus).
4. Count both sides of chamber and average counts of both sides (4 sq mm area).
5. Apply formula: (#WBC counted/area counted × fluid depth) × dilution.

For the <u>differential count</u>, prepare a blood smear, stain the smear, examine with microscope under oil immersion objective, and count each cell until 100 cells counted, noting any abnormalities. Note blast or immature cells. Nucleated red blood cells observed are counted separately.

SOURCES OF ERROR AND CORRECTIVE ACTIONS FOR PLATELET COUNTS

Platelet counts (150,000-450,000) are usually done electronically, but the tendency of platelets to clump and their small size can interfere with accurate counts. Accuracy decreases with low platelet numbers (around 100,000), sometimes causing analyzers to overestimate the counts by up to 30%. Abnormal findings:

- <u>Falsely decreased counts</u> may result from inadequate anticoagulation, platelet clumping, presence of giant platelets, and platelet adherence to neutrophils (satellitism resulting from antibodies). The solution may be to use a fresh fingerstick sample for a blood film. Manual counting may be necessary for giant platelets, which may be miscounted as RBCs. For platelet aggregation caused by EDTA, solutions include adding more EDTA, adding kanamycin (20 mg), collecting a sample in citrate rather than EDTA, or using a fingerstick sample with no anticoagulant.
- <u>Falsely elevated counts</u> may result from microcytosis, fragmentation of leukocytes, and presence of cryoglobulins. The solution may be to do a phase contrast microscopic examination or estimation based on a blood film. All abnormal counts should be confirmed with a second test.

BODY FLUID ANALYSIS, COUNTS, AND RELATED MORPHOLOGY

Cerebrospinal fluid is similar to plasma, from which it is derived, but with lower levels of protein and some electrolyte differences. Composition:

Appearance: clear with no clot	Protein: Myelin basic—<4.0 ng/mL, IgG—3.4 mg/dL
Electrolytes: Na 138 mEq/L, K 2.8 mEq/L, Ca, 2.1 mEq/L, Mg 2-2.5 mEq/L, Cl 119 mEq/L	WBC count: 0-1 mo.—0-30 cells/mm^3, 5-adult—0-5 cells/mm^3. No abnormal cells. RBC count: 0
Glucose: Infant/child—60-80 mg/dL, Adult—40-70 mg/dL.	Lactic acid: Neonate—10-60 mg/dL, Adult—<25.2 mg/dL

Synovial fluid composition:

Appearance: clear to pale yellow, viscous. No crystals.	Protein: <3 g/dL.
Glucose: <10 mg/dL.	WBC count: <200/mm^3. No abnormal cells/inclusions. Granulocytes <25%. RBC count: 0

Results for ANA, C3, uric acid, and RF for synovial fluid should be similar to results for serum.

Serous fluid is found in body cavities. Transudates result from impaired regulation of fluid balance, which causes fluid to leak from capillaries while exudates result from disorders of the surrounding membrane, such as cancer or infection, which allows larger molecules to leak through blood vessels.

Peritoneal /Pleural fluids	Transudate	Exudate
Appearance	Clear, watery	Cloudy
Sp. gravity	<1.015	>1.018
Protein	<2.5 g/dL	2.9 g/dL
Odor	None	Odor if infection present
Glucose	10-20 mg/dL	Very low
White blood cell count	<100 cells/mm^3	>1000 cells/mm^3
Red blood cell count	<1000 cells/mm^3	Varies
pH	7.60-7.64	<7.3
Pleural fluid to serum protein ratio	<0.5	>0.5
Pleural fluid to serum LDH ratio	<0.6	>0.6

SEMEN ANALYSIS

Semen analysis is done to diagnose fertility problems. The sample of ejaculate should be transported at body temperature in a clean glass container for examination. A fresh sample at testing sight is preferable. A condom should not be used for collection. Semen is white/opaque and viscous with a distinctive musty odor. Composition:

- pH: 7.2-8.0
- Volume: 2-5 mL, <1.5 mL is abnormal.
- Clotting/Liquefaction: Usually complete in 15 to 20 minutes. Should complete within 30 minutes.
- Sperm count: >15 million/mL.
- Total sperm count: >39 million per ejaculation.
- Motility at 60 minutes: ≥40%.
- Vitality: ≥60%.
- Morphology: >25%-30% (preferably >70%) normal in appearance. Appearance: 50-70 µm in length with large oval head, slender tail (90% of length), and small neck.

Abnormalities that may require further testing include decreased sperm count and decreased motility. Sperm count decreased: hyperpyrexia, ejaculatory obstruction, orchitis, testicular failure/atrophy, varicocele, and post-vasectomy.

SOURCES OF ERROR IN HEMATOLOGICAL TESTS

Sources of **errors in hematological tests** include instrumentation errors (most common) and personal errors, most often associated with a failure to follow standard protocols:

- Use of incorrect collection tube: Follow protocol and check requirements.
- Hemolysis: Ensure proper collection, mixing, and storing of blood samples.
- Incorrectly calibrated equipment: Follow manufacturer's guidelines and lab protocols.
- Incorrectly prepared thin and thick blood films: Check film and redo if problems occur.
- Dirty/defective equipment: Check all equipment before use.

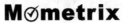

- Inaccurate use of equipment: Check directions for use if unsure or unfamiliar with equipment.
- Improper technique: Follow established protocols every time.
- Outdated reagent: Check dates and rotate supply.
- Sample degraded: Process samples within prescribed time period.
- Inaccurate cell counting: Make sure to be alert and exercise care.
- Anticoagulant concentration too high: Adjust for high hematocrit levels.
- Incorrect mixing of sample: Follow standard procedure, mix properly, avoiding excessive shaking.

MOLECULAR ASSAYS

Molecular assays, such as PCR-ELISA and fluorescence in situ hybridization, are able to detect molecules or specific sequences in the genetic code that are markers for specific disease processes. Assays may be qualitative or quantitative. Molecular assays, which require a blood or stool sample, are less invasive than biopsies. Tests utilize RNA or DNA to determine if there are abnormalities causing disease. Assays can be designed about specific drug targets or receptors and are important in development of drugs. A biochemical assay uses DNA to monitor chemical reactions. A functional assay measures a physiological response to a drug. During a molecular assay, nucleic acid is extracted and purified and then amplified to make multiple copies. Commercial molecular assays are approved by the FDA. CLIA establishes standards and requirements for laboratory-developed assays, which are often used for patient management. Molecular assays may be used to diagnose different types of malignancies, infections, genetic disorders, coagulation disorders, and HLA typing.

CBC AND DIFFERENTIAL USING AUTOMATED HEMATOLOGY INSTRUMENTATION

Automated analyzers carry out the CBC and differential. Some analyzers are small and process one blood sample at a time. A sample is mixed and a small amount aspirated into the machine. Others are able to process dozens of samples, which are labeled and placed in special racks. Technology utilized in analyzers includes:

- Impedance analysis: Blood passes in a one-cell diameter stream through electrodes that pass a charge through the blood cells according to the cell size, allowing the analyzer to act as a cell counter able to count thousands of cells each second. The analyzer is able to differentiate and count RBCs, lymphocytes, and monocytes, but can only count total granulocytes, not differentiate them.
- Laser flow cytometry: Similar to impedance analysis except the stream passes through lasers, which measure absorbance, and are able to better differentiate cell morphology for the WBC differential.
- Fluorescent flow cytometry: Adds fluorescent reagents to show the ratio of nucleus to plasma for each cell in order to count platelets, reticulocytes, and nucleated RBCs.

STAINS RELATED TO HEMATOLOGY

1. Nonvital polychrome stains: also known as Romanowsky stains; DNA and RNA turn blue, acid components turn orange or red, red blood cells turn pink
2. Nonvital monochrome stains: used to stay in histocytes, iron granules, and other particular cellular parts in a red blood cell; Prussian blue is a common example
3. Vital monochrome stains: used to stay in the nature to hemoglobin and other specific cellular parts; Heinz body stains and reticulocyte stains are two common examples

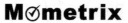

NORMAL HISTOGRAM FOR ERYTHROCYTES, LEUKOCYTES, AND PLATELETS

A normal erythrocyte histogram will be between 36 and 360 femtoliters, with a peak representing mean corpuscular volume between 70 and 110. A normal leukocyte histogram, meanwhile, will be between 45 and 450 fL, with the three peaks. The first peak, 45 to 90 fL, is the normal range of lymphocytes; the second peak, 90 to 160 fL, is the normal range for immature leukocytes and monocytes; the third peak, 160 to 450 fL, is the normal range for granulocytes. A normal thrombocyte histogram will be between 2 and 20 femtoliters, and will not have any peaks.

ABNORMAL HISTOGRAM FOR ERYTHROCYTES AND LEUKOCYTES

If the curve on a red blood cell histogram is especially wide, it may be that there has been an elevation in the red blood cell distribution width. If the red blood cell histogram has two peaks, this may be an indication of the presence of both microcytic and macrocytic erythrocytes. A shift to the left or to the right indicates a decrease or increase, respectively, in mean corpuscular volume. As for white blood cell histograms, an overlap of peaks at approximately 90 fL may indicate an elevated number of immature cells or bands, while values over 450 fL may indicate a high granulocyte count. Values lower than 50 fL suggest the existence of nucleated red blood cells, sickle cells, or large clumps of platelets.

NECESSARY PRECAUTIONS/PROCEDURES WHEN COLLECTING, HANDLING, AND PROCESSING SAMPLES FOR COAGULATION TESTING

Lab technicians need to be especially careful when handling, collecting, and processing coagulation test samples. The drawing of the blood should be nontraumatic, so that coagulation is not activated. Samples should be placed into silicon-coated glass tubes or plastic tubes; the use of glass tubes without silicon coating may activate factors XI, XII, and prekallikrein. Samples must contain a sufficient amount of blood and must be processed within two hours. All testing must be performed at a temperature of 37°C, lest factors VII and XI be activated by cold temperatures or factors V and VIII break down at room temperature.

POSSIBLE SOURCES OF ERROR WHEN MANUALLY COUNTING BLOOD CELLS

Lab technicians must guard against several kinds of common error when manually counting blood cells. Equipment that is not properly cleaned and dried may contribute to counting errors. A failure to dilute samples appropriately or follow the correct procedures in counting may lead to error. If the sample is not maintained at the appropriate temperature, it may develop clots, which will skew the count.

CYTOCHEMICAL STAINING

Cytochemical staining is used to identify enzymes, cell type, or other substances in blood cell cytoplasm based on color reactions to a reagent. The purpose is to identify cells; diagnose, differentiate, and/or confirm diagnosis of leukemia; identify enzyme deficiencies; and detect abnormalities of cytoplasm. Cytochemical staining includes an enzyme plus a substrate (substance with which the enzyme will react) leading to an identifiable color change. Chemical stains may be enzymatic (myeloperoxidase, non-specific esterase, specific esterase, and tartrate-resistance acid phosphatase) or non-enzymatic (toluidine blue, PAS, Sudan black). The procedure will vary somewhat depending on the chemical stain utilized. Basic procedure:

1. Fix a smear (air dried) with the appropriate fixative (such as cold buffered acetone or formalin vapors) for the prescribed period, ranging from seconds to 10-15 minutes.
2. Process and stain the smear through various steps:
3. Rinse with water or air wash for prescribed period of time.
4. Incubate in substrate solution if required.

87

5. Wash and stain as needed.
6. Counterstain as needed.
7. Rinse and air dry if needed.
8. Note results and reaction product.

PREPARING/STAIN PERIPHERAL BLOOD SMEAR AND BONE MARROW SLIDES AND CORRELATING WITH CBC

Thin films for **blood smears and bone marrow smears** are the best choice for assessing the morphology of blood cells and verifying cell counts. Blood smears are often done when the results of the CBC were abnormal to check all 3 cells lines. Procedure:

1. Transfer 4 mm diameter drop of EDTA-anticoagulated blood or bone marrow aspirant to end of one slide.
2. Position a spreader slide at a 45° angle just ahead of the drop.
3. Pull to spreader along the slide until it touches the drop.
4. Allow the drop to spread along the spreader edge.
5. Push the spreader to the other end of the slide, keeping the 45° angle, drawing the blood along the slide.
6. Wave the slide to thoroughly dry blood.
7. Stain (Wright or Wright-Giemsa) by flooding slide, drying for 3 minutes or more, and then rising with distilled/non-ionized water and air drying.

If streaks or lines are evident along the slide, the blood was clotting. Bone marrow smears are usually compared to a blood smear.

PREPARING SLIDES AND EVALUATING FOR IDENTIFICATION OF MALARIAL PARASITES

Preparing slides and evaluating for **identification of malarial parasites** (*Plasmodium* spp.):

- Gather supplies: microscope, slides, slide spreaders, containers for Field stain, draining racks, applicator sticks.
- Obtain blood specimen (anticoagulated venous blood or non-anticoagulated capillary blood).
- Place one drop of blood on slide for a thin film to identify species and RBC morphology. Spread blood with spreader at ≤45° angle.
- Place 2-3 drops of blood on slide for thick film to detect density. Spread blood evenly over about a 1 cm area (should be translucent while wet).
- Label films and allow to dry for at least 30 minutes.
- Fix the thin film with methanol but not the thick. Stain thin film with Giemsa and thick with Field stain.
- Air dry.
- Examine under high-powered microscope and oil immersion.

Use thick film to determine density of parasites. *P. falciparum* has high density; *P. vivax,* medium, and *P. malariae,* low. Use thin film to identify the stages of the parasite (trophozoites, schizont, gametocyte). The RBCs are no longer visible but pink Schüffner's dots appear about parasites and trophozoite cytoplasm stains blue.

USE OF STAINS IN THE LABORATORY

Crystal violet can be used in the laboratory to determine the presence of Heinz bodies in red blood cells (erythrocytes). Prussian blue can be used to detect iron in bone marrow, peripheral blood, or

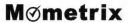

in urine. Sudan black B is used to determine the presence of lipids (fats), and Wright's stain can be used to determine the presence of basophilic stippling. Howell-Jolly bodies, and Pappenheimer bodies.

COMPLETE BLOOD CELL COUNT EXAMPLES

A non-pregnant, adult female comes into the laboratory for a complete blood cell count to be performed. List the results that you would expect if the woman was healthy.

A non-pregnant, adult female who is healthy should expect to have the following results in her complete blood count (CBC): Red blood cell (RBC) count of 4.2—5.0 million/microliter, white blood cell (WBC) count of 4,500—11,000/microliter, hematocrit of 35—47%, hemoglobin of 12—15 g/dL, and a platelet count of 150,000—400,000/microliter. The white blood cell differential should show the following breakdown of white blood cells: 50—70% neutrophils, 1—3% eosinophils, 0.4—1% basophils, 25—35% lymphocytes, 4—6% monocytes, and 0—5% bands. The red blood cell indices in a non-pregnant, healthy, adult female should be: Mean cell volume (MCV) of 80—98 femtoliters, mean cell hemoglobin (MCH) of 27—31 picograms, mean cell hemoglobin concentration (MCHC) of 32-36%, and red cell distribution width of 11.5—14.5%.

An adult with macrocytic anemia comes into the laboratory. Describe, in general terms, how the values in his/her complete blood cell count (CBC) should vary from normal values.

Macrocytic anemia is a disorder in which the red blood cells present in a person's blood are larger than they should be because they lack folic acid. These large red blood cells are called macrocytes, and will appear on the blood smear. The patient will also have a low hemoglobin value, low hematocrit, and a low red blood cell count. The mean cell volume (MCV) will be higher than normal. Folic acid deficiency in pregnant women leads to spina bifida in the fetus.

RELATIVE ANEMIA OF PREGNANCY

Relative anemia occurs during the third trimester of pregnancy. It is a mild condition featuring slightly lowered hemoglobin, and often these women have normal iron levels in their blood. However, relative anemia of pregnancy can also be found in pregnant women that do have an iron deficiency. Relative anemia of pregnancy is caused by the rapidly increasing amount of plasma during pregnancy (doubled blood volume). Red blood cell count also increases during pregnancy, but the amount of plasma increases at a higher rate. Therefore, this causes an increased blood volume and a relative anemia. Relative anemia of pregnancy, however, does increase the movement of oxygen to both the fetus and the mother. There are no permanent negative health effects; the problem resolves after birth.

APLASTIC ANEMIA

Aplastic anemia is a disorder in which the bone marrow does not produce enough erythrocytes (red blood cells), leukocytes (white blood cells), and platelets. This disease can be caused by an autoimmune disorder, or by exposure to certain chemicals, drugs, or radiation. However, approximately half of all cases have no known cause. Because of the decreased amount of granulocytes, patients with aplastic anemia are susceptible to infections. And, because of the abnormally low amount of platelets produced, hemorrhaging, prolonged PT/PTT, and bruising are often seen. The disease is ultimately diagnosed by a bone marrow biopsy, and the best course of treatment is a bone marrow transplant.

SIDEROBLASTIC ANEMIA

Sideroblastic anemia is a disease that is characterized by sideroblasts in the bone marrow. A sideroblast is a nucleated erythroblast that contains granules of ferritin. Because of the ferritin contained in the sideroblasts, patients with sideroblastic anemia have higher than normal ferritin levels, as well as a decrease in the ability to bind total iron (TIBC). Normal groups of red blood cells exist in the patient's bone marrow, alongside the sideroblasts. Sideroblastic anemia can be both genetic and acquired. Genetic sideroblastic anemia is a sex-linked disorder, and is seen most often in males. However, the acquired form of the disease is seen in both males and females.

SICKLE CELL TRAIT VS. SICKLE CELL DISEASE

Patients with sickle cell trait have inherited from their parents one abnormal hemoglobin gene, hemoglobin S. Hemoglobin S is responsible for turning red blood cells into abnormal sickle shaped (curved) cells. Patients with sickle cell trait, however, also have one gene for normal hemoglobin, hemoglobin A. Because these patients do have some hemoglobin A, they rarely exhibit any adverse symptoms. However, they can pass the sickle cell trait onto their children. Patients with sickle cell disease, on the other hand, have inherited two genes for hemoglobin S, and no genes for hemoglobin A. Therefore, the latter will exhibit the adverse symptoms of the disease, like severely debilitating joint pain during sickle cell crisis. They also will pass the gene for hemoglobin S onto any children they may have (who may or may not develop sickle cell disease).

LEUKOCYTE DISORDERS CORRELATED WITH WBC DIFFERENTIAL

Differential	Normal	Changes
Total WBC	4,800-10,000	Increased (10,000+): Severe infection. (See differential for other.) Decreased (<4000): Viral infection, autoimmune disorders.
Total neutrophils	2.7-6.5 4.5-11.1%	Increased: Infections, injuries, inflammatory disorders, lymphocytic leukemias. Decreased: Bacterial infections, viral infections, aplastic anemia, autoimmune disorders, splenomegaly, chemotherapy, toxin exposure.
Immature neutrophils (bands)	0.1-0.3 1-3%	Increased: Infection, acute hemorrhage, acute hemolysis, malignancies, metabolic disorders, myelocytic leukemia, tissue necrosis, toxin ingestion. Decreased: Addison disease, anaphylaxis, anorexia nervosa, SLE, viral infection, folate deficiency, thyrotoxicosis.
Segmented neutrophils	2.5-6.2 50-62%	Increased: Acute, localized, or systemic bacterial infections.
Eosinophils	0.05-0.5 0-3%	Decreased: Stress and acute infection.
Basophils	0-0.1 0-1%	Decreased: Acute stage of infection.
Lymphocytes	1.5-3.7 25-40%	Increased: Some viral and bacterial infections, Addison disease, lymphocytic leukemia, lymphomas, myeloma, lymphosarcoma, ulcerative colitis. Decreased: Burns, Hodgkin disease, pernicious anemia, radiation, septicemia, corticosteroids, bone marrow failure, immunosuppressive drugs, thrombocytopenia purpura, transfusion reaction.
Monocytes	0.2-0.4 3-7%	Increased: Recovery stage of acute infection, cirrhosis, hemolytic anemias, Hodgkin disease, sarcoidosis, radiation, polycythemia vera, collagen diseases.

ACUTE LEUKEMIA VS. CHRONIC LEUKEMIA

Acute leukemias are characterized by an extremely rapid growth of immature white blood cells (leukocytes) in the bone marrow. These new cells are unable to kill invaders because of their immaturity. Immature leukocytes may crowd out normal leukocytes in the bone marrow. Acute leukemias occur most often in young adults and children. Acute leukemias progress very rapidly, and so treatment of the disease needs to be started immediately after diagnosis. Chronic leukemias, on the other hand, are characterized by the growth of abnormal (but relatively mature) leukocytes. The abnormal leukocytes are produced at a higher rate than the production of normal leukocytes in the bone marrow. This disease can take a long time to progress, on the order of months to even years. Chronic leukemia is most commonly found in the elderly, and unlike with acute leukemias, treatment does not need to begin immediately after diagnosis, because chronic leukemias do not progress very rapidly.

HAIRY CELL LEUKEMIA

Hairy cell leukemia is a rare, chronic disease that is characterized by the presence of hairy cells in the bone marrow. Hairy cells are leukocytes (white blood cells) that have hair like projections. They are found in the bone marrow, the spleen, and in some cases, the liver. B-lymphocytes are the most often affected by this type of leukemia. Hairy cell leukemia occurs most often in the elderly, and is often associated with enlargement of the spleen. Some symptoms of hairy cell leukemia include: Fatigue, excessive bruising, abdominal pain, infections, and anemia. The cause of hairy cell leukemia is unknown, but there may be a genetic component to the disease. In the laboratory, when hairy cells are exposed to acid phosphatase, they stain positive. When they are exposed to tartaric acid, however, they do not destain.

BASOPHILIC STIPPLING, HEINZ BODIES, HOWELL-JOLLY BODIES, ROULEAUX, AND SCHISTOCYTES

Basophilic stippling could be seen in a patient with lead poisoning. Heinz bodies are characteristic of hemolytic anemia, and Howell-Jolly bodies are characteristic of megaloblastic anemia. Rouleaux of erythrocytes is seen in patients with myeloma, and schistocytes can be seen in patients that have high blood pressure (hypertension).

HEMOLYTIC DISEASE OF THE NEWBORN (HDN)

Hemolytic disease of the newborn (HDN) occurs when IgG antibodies are produced by the mother and then transferred through the placenta to her developing fetus. IgG antibodies attack the fetus's red blood cells, causing jaundice or anemia at birth. The effects on the fetus can be severe enough to require blood transfusions in the womb, usually if the mother has been sensitized during a previous full-term pregnancy or therapeutic abortion. Hemolytic disease of the newborn is caused when: The mother receives a blood transfusion that is incompatible with her own blood type; or the mother has negative blood, and the father and fetus have positive blood; or placental rupture or uterine trauma occurs during pregnancy; or the mother with O blood type produces IgG antibodies to the A and B antigens present in her environment, and these cross the placenta to the fetus.

HEMOGLOBIN H DISEASE

Hemoglobin H disease is an inherited, genetic disorder also known as alpha thalassemia major. It is common among Mediterranean peoples. Patients with thalassemia tend to have a moderate form of anemia caused by the defective production of hemoglobin. In hemoglobin H disease, several of the genes (usually three or four genes) that regulate the production of alpha globin chains are missing. This leads to a decrease in the production of alpha globin chains, and a corresponding increase in the production of beta chains. The defective hemoglobin that is formed is called hemoglobin H.

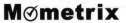

Hemoglobin H is highly attracted to oxygen, but it is an unstable molecule. Therefore, red blood cells containing hemoglobin H have a shorter life span than cells containing normal hemoglobin A.

PICA

Pica is a disorder in which a person consumes non-food items (e.g., clay, coal, chalk, body mucus), or consumes some food items inappropriately, such as raw flour, or ice. In order for a person to be diagnosed with pica, these abnormal eating habits must persist for at least a month. In children, pica is associated with lead poisoning. Children who consume old paint that contains lead from their home, contaminated soil, or lead paint on their toys or other household objects, develop lead poisoning as a result of their pica. In adults, pica is associated with a mineral deficiency, such as anemics who lack iron and eat ice. Often, adults will not eat items that contain the mineral that they are lacking. If the deficiency is treated medically, then the pica usually ceases.

HODGKIN'S DISEASE

Hodgkin's disease is a type of lymphoma in which cells in the lymphatic system grow abnormally. The disease usually starts in a neck or chest lymph node and then it spreads throughout the body in a predictable pattern. The spleen, liver, and lymph nodes enlarge. Hodgkin's disease is most common in older adults (in their 50s) and in young adults (late teens to late twenties), and it is more common in males than in females. The Rye classification system is used to describe the disease. The causes of Hodgkin's disease are not known, and it can be fatal, although the cure rate is 93%. Biopsy the swollen lymph nodes and look for the presence of Reed-Sternberg cells, giant lymphocytes that have more than one nucleus (polynuclear). Other types of lymphomas do not show the tell-tale Reed-Sternberg cells present in Hodgkin's disease.

GAUCHER'S DISEASE

Gaucher's disease is a genetic disease characterized by the abnormal storage of lipids. People with this particular disease lack an enzyme, beta-glucosidase, which is used to break down lipids in the body Without this enzyme, there is a harmful buildup of lipids (glycosphingolipids) in the liver, spleen, brain, bone marrow, and joints, which destroys the tissues. Patients have brownish skin with bruising, ascites, and yellowed sclera of the eyes. Some side effects of Gaucher's disease include anemia, low platelet count, spleen enlargement, and various neurological complications. There are three types of Gaucher's disease. Type I occurs among Ashkenazi Jews and patients live to adulthood. Type II develops within six months after birth, and is always fatal by early toddlerhood (age 2-3). Type III is chronic, and patients live to be teenagers.

CHRONIC GRANULOMATOUS DISEASE (CGD)

Chronic granulomatous disease (CGD) is a hereditary, X-linked disease in which phagocytes cannot kill pathogens. Mostly boys under 10 years old are affected, and will likely die by the age of 30. Phagocytes cannot produce superoxide anions to destroy invaders because they lack NADPH oxidase. Therefore, a patient with chronic granulomatous disease has recurrent fungal and bacterial infections, which can be fatal. This lack of NADPH enzyme also allows for oxidative products, such as hydrogen peroxide, to build up and cause death. In the laboratory, the nitroblue tetrazolium test can be used to determine the existence of chronic granulomatous disease. Patients with CGD will have neutrophils with greatly reduced nitroblue tetrazolium activity.

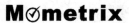

MOLECULAR ASSAYS RELEVANT TO THE DIAGNOSIS OF HEMATOLOGIC NEOPLASMS

Molecular assays relevant to the diagnosis of hematologic neoplasms include:

Genetic tests:

- Karyotyping (G-band metaphase chromosome analysis): Identifies translocations and other chromosomal abnormalities.
- FISH (fluorescence in situ hybridization): Utilizes fluorescently labeled DNA probes to find abnormalities.

MICROARRAY TECHNIQUES:

- Whole genome scanning by comparative genomic hybridization: Compares genetic material with pooled DNA that represents a normal individual.
- Molecular karyotyping (SNP arrays): Used to identify genetic deletions and copy number aberrations.
- Profiling of gene expression: Measures activities of genes.

PCR TECHNIQUES:

- Reverse transcription/Reverse transcription quantitative real-time PCR: Uses RNA or cDNA to identify chromosomal translocations.
- Multiplex ligation probe amplification (MLPA): Used to detect mutations.
- Fragment analysis: Used to identify mutations and products based on size, similar to electrophoresis.

SEQUENCING TECHNIQUES:

- Pyrosequencing: Used to identify mutations (if allele percentage >10% to 20%).

POSSIBLE CAUSES FOR VARIOUS CONDITIONS

1. Neutrophilia: neutrophils count is increased, probably because of inflammation, leukemia, exercise, bacterial infection, or inflammation
2. Neutropenia: neutrophil count is decreased, probably because of damaged spleen, vitamin B12 or folate deficiency, or infection
3. Eosinophilia: eosinophil count is increased, probably because of scarlet fever, hay fever, parasitic infection, hives, asthma, or chronic myelocytic leukemia
4. Eosinopenia: eosinophil count is decreased, probably because of high stress or acute inflammation
5. Basophilia: basophil count is increased, probably because of hypothyroidism, chronic hemolytic anemia, hypersensitivity reaction, or another myeloproliferative disorder
6. Basopenia: basophile count is decreased, probably because of infection or hypothyroidism

APPEARANCE OF ATYPICAL LYMPHOCYTES

Atypical lymphocytes are larger in size than normal lymphocytes, and typically have less nucleus relative to cytoplasm. The cytoplasm in an atypical lymphocyte is dark blue, owing to elevated production of RNA. Nucleoli will be visible, and the Golgi apparatus will be larger than usual. A distinctive transparent area in the Golgi apparatus, known as the Hof area, will appear under the microscope.

VARIOUS LEUKEMIAS OR LYMPHOMAS

1. Philadelphia chromosome: also known as Ph1 chromosome; associated with chronic myelocytic leukemia, adult T-cell leukemia, and acute lymphocytic leukemia
2. Reed-Sternberg cells: associated with Hodgkin's lymphoma
3. Howell-Jolly bodies: associated with acute be erythroleukemia; these bodies are small and round, and are found in the nuclei of red blood cells

THALASSEMIA

Thalassemia is a condition in which there is a deficiency in the synthesis of at least one globin chain in the hemoglobin molecule. Thalassemia major is a condition in which there are neither alpha nor beta globin chains in the hemoglobin, while thalassemia minor is a condition in which there are simply decreased amounts of alpha and beta globin chains. The standard test for diagnosing this condition is hemoglobin electrophoresis. If the test shows increased fetal hemoglobin and Hb A_2, then thalassemia is indicated.

PORPHYRIA

In the condition known as porphyria, an individual has a diminished production of heme resulting from an enzyme deficiency. Such individuals may manifest microcytic or hypo-chronic anemia, and will display decreased mean corpuscular volume, mean corpuscular hemoglobin, and mean corpuscular hemoglobin concentration. Abdominal pain, sensitivity to light, and disorders of the central nervous system are common symptoms. This condition may be either inherited or acquired. Two examples of inherited porphyrias are erythrohepatic protoporphyria and acute intermittent porphyria. One example of an acquired porphyria is porphyria cutanea.

PLATELET DISORDERS

1. Thrombocytopenia: decrease in the production of platelets; may be the result of ineffective thrombopoiesis, loss of platelets due to hemorrhage or hemolytic uremic syndrome, spleen conditions, or megakaryocyte hypoproliferation
2. Primary thrombocytosis: wild elevation in the production of platelets; may be caused by chronic granulocytic leukemia, polycythemia vera, or essential thrombocythemia
3. Secondary thrombocytosis: increase in the production of platelets, slightly less than that of primary thrombocytosis; often caused by chronic inflammatory disease, acute inflammatory disease, acute blood loss, iron deficiency, hemolytic anemia, or malignant disease

Coagulation and Hemostasis

HEMOSTASIS

Hemostasis is the cessation of bleeding. There are four main steps involved in hemostasis: 1. A damaged blood vessel narrows (vasoconstriction) and the reduced diameter helps slow down any bleeding. 2. Platelets that are present in the blood attach themselves to the collagen in the walls of the blood vessel to create a hemostatic plug within seconds. This process is sometimes referred to as primary hemostasis. After the formation of a hemostatic plug, secondary hemostasis occurs. The clotting factors help fibrin form from fibrinogen. The fibrin then aids in the formation of blood clot at the wound site. Secondary hemostasis takes a few minutes. 3. The newly-formed blood clot helps the wound site create new smooth muscle cells to repair the wound. The clot can then be lyzed (destroyed) when it is not needed any longer.

PLATELETS

A platelet is a cell fragment is derived from a megakaryocyte. Platelets form in bone marrow, are stored in the spleen, and then move to blood plasma to assist with blood clotting after an injury. Platelets are small, colorless, and irregularly shaped. They have no hemoglobin, no nucleus, and no DNA. Platelets also transport and store several chemicals. A normal platelet count for a healthy adult is between 150,000 and 400,000 per microliter of blood. Platelets are also called thrombocytes.

COAGULATION TERMINOLOGY

Coagulation	Formation of a clot. Four stage process: (1) damaged vessel constricts; (2) platelets adhere to damaged area (platelet adhesion) to form a platelet plug; (3) Extrinsic and intrinsic pathways lead to common pathway in which prothrombin activator reacts with calcium ions to form prothrombin, which forms thrombin, which causes fibrinogen to form fibrin monomers that react with fibrin stabilizing factor and calcium ions to form fibrin polymers that attract platelets and phospholipids to form a clot; (4) Fibrinolysis (clot breakdown) occurs when plasmin breaks fibrin into fragments, which are then removed by phagocytes
Sodium citrate	Anticoagulant (crystalline compound) that prevents clotting but preserves coagulation factors.
Thrombin	Clot activator that converts fibrinogen into fibrin.
Platelet function test	Tests the ability of platelets to form a clot and helps to diagnose bleeding disorders.
Warfarin (Coumadin®)	Warfarin (Coumadin®) is an anticoagulant that interferes with the formation of vitamin K–associated clotting factors (II, VII, IX, X) and C and S anticoagulant proteins.

FIBRIN

Fibrin: Fibrin is a protein that aids in blood clotting. Along with platelets, fibrin helps form blood clots. Fibrin is made from the glycoprotein fibrinogen, in the liver.

HEPARIN

Heparin: Heparin is a polysaccharide anticoagulant that helps prevent blood clotting. Heparin is concentrated in the vessels surrounding the liver and the lungs. It can also be found in the spleen

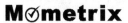

and various other muscles. Heparin is also a drug that can be given to patients that need to take advantage of its anticoagulant properties, such as in the case of a pulmonary embolism.

PLASMIN

Plasmin: Plasmin is an enzyme that helps dissolve (lyze) fibrin that is present in blood clots. Lyzing a clot turns coagulated blood into liquid blood again. Plasmin is derived from plasminogen in the blood plasma.

HEMOPHILIA

Hemophilia is an inherited disease in which the body has trouble forming blood clots because it lacks a clotting factor. People afflicted with hemophilia have the tendency to hemorrhage and have episodes of uncontrolled bleeding. The bleeding can either be external or internal. Hemophilia is a sex-linked disease (recessive on the X chromosome), and because of this, males are more likely to be hemophiliacs than are female's. Many royal families in Europe inherited hemophilia from Queen Victoria. Hemophilia is passed from mother (the carrier) to son. There are three types of hemophilia, A, B, and C. These types are all defined by a different deficiency in a clotting factor necessary for the formation of blood clots and for the control of bleeding.

ADJUSTING ANTICOAGULANT-TO-BLOOD RATIO

Anticoagulant-blood ratio adjustment: If a patient's hematocrit is higher than 55%, it is more viscous than normal and contains a lower percentage of plasma. Because of this, for samples collected in a tube with anticoagulant, such as sodium citrate, centrifugation will result in plasma with an increased level of anticoagulant. This, in turn, can affect the test results for all tests run on the sample, so a second sample with anticoagulant corrected should be obtained. For example, a formula is applied to determine the amount of sodium citrate to remove from a tube. For calculation, a 5-mL tube contains 4.5 mL of blood; a 3-mL tube, 2.7 mL; and a 2 mL, 1.8 mL. The volume of sodium citrate for 5-mL tube is 0.5 mL, for the 3-mL tube is 0.3 mL, and for the 2-mL tube is 0.2 mL:

- Sodium citrate volume = $(1.85 \times 10)^{-3} \times (100 - \text{hematocrit}) \times \text{volume of blood}$

Once the volume needed is determined, then the excess anticoagulant is removed from the tube before the blood draw. Correction charts are also available for the various tube sizes. For 5 mL (4.5 mL) tube:

Hematocrit	Sodium citrate volume
57	0.36 mL
63	0.31 mL

PRINCIPLE BEHIND THE PLATELET AGGREGOMETER

The platelet aggregometer measures platelet aggregation, when platelets attach to each other to form a clot. Add a coagulation agent, such as ADP, epinephrine, or collagen, to a sample of plasma that showed a high concentration of platelets in the Coulter Counter during the automated CBC. Place the mixture into the aggregometer. The plasma is initially optically dense. As the platelets start to aggregate, the plasma becomes clearer until only serum and the clot remain. In other words, the plasma, with increasing aggregation of platelets, gains the ability to transmit light.

MOLECULAR TESTING AND MOLECULAR ASSAYS IN COAGULATION

Molecular testing and molecular assays are used in coagulation studies because they have increased specificity as well as increased sensitivity, and testing can be carried out while the patient is receiving anticoagulant medications. Molecular testing is especially useful for inherited diseases because many coagulation disorders (factor V Leiden mutation, hyperhomocysteinemia, and prothrombin 20210 G>A mutation) and bleeding disorders (hemophilia A and B, von Willebrand disease) involve molecular defects. However, in some cases molecular testing is not practical because of numerous possible mutations, such as with antithrombin testing and protein C and S deficiencies. Numerous different types of procedure are utilized, but one of the most common is the PCR-based assay, especially for inherited clotting disorders, with restriction fragment length polymorphism analysis or other methods. A number of direct hybridization methods, such as the Invader assay, are also available.

COAGULATION PROCEDURES

Prothrombin time (PT)	10–14 seconds	Collect 1 mL blood in sodium citrate blue-capped tube (completely filled). Increased: Anticoagulation therapy, vitamin K deficiency, decreased prothrombin, DIC, liver disease, and malignant neoplasm. Some drugs may shorten time.
Partial thromboplastin time (PTT)	30–45 seconds	Collect 1 mL blood in sodium citrate blue-capped tube (completely filled). Increased: hemophilia A & B, von Willebrand disease, vitamin deficiency, lupus, DIC, and liver disease.
Activated partial thromboplastin time (aPTT)	21–35 seconds	Collect 1 mL blood in sodium citrate blue-capped tube (completely filled). Similar to PTT but an activator added that speeds clotting time. Used to monitor heparin dosage. Increased: See PTT. Decreased: Extensive cancer, early DIC, and after acute hemorrhage.
D-dimer	0.5 mcg/mL FEU*	Collect 1 mL blood in sodium citrate blue-capped tube (completely filled) for immunoturbidimetry. Transport frozen.
		D-dimer is a specific polymer that results when fibrin breaks down, giving a marker to indicate the degree of fibrinolysis. Increased: DIC, pulmonary embolism, DVT, late pregnancy, neoplastic disorder, preeclampsia, arterial/venous thrombosis.
Fibrinogen (factor I)	100-400 mg/dL	Collect 1 mL blood in sodium citrate blue-capped tube (completely filled) for photo-optical clot detection.
		Synthesized in liver, converts to fibrin, which combines with platelets in coagulation sequence. Increased: Acute MI, cancer, eclampsia, multiple myeloma, Hodgkin disease, nephrotic syndrome, tissue trauma. Decreased: DIC, liver disease, congenital fibrinogen abnormality.

Fibrin degradation product (fibrin split products [FSPs])	<5 mcg/mL FEU	Collect 1 mL blood in sodium citrate blue-capped tube (completely filled) for latex agglutination test. Transport frozen. FSPs occur as clots form and more breakdown of fibrinogen and fibrin occurs, interfering with blood coagulation by coating platelets and disrupting thrombin, and attaching to fibrinogen so stable clots can't form. Increased: DIC, liver disease, MI, hemorrhage, pulmonary embolism, renal disease, obstetric complications, kidney transplant rejection.
Heparin assay (antithrombin III)	1-3 mo: 48-108%	Collect 1 mL blood in sodium citrate blue-capped tube (completely filled) for chromogenic immunoturbidimetry. Utilized to diagnose heparin resistance in patients receiving heparin therapy and to diagnose hypercoagulable conditions. Increased: Acute hepatitis, kidney transplantation, vitamin K deficiency. Decreased: DIC, liver transplantation, nephrotic syndrome, pulmonary embolism, venous thrombosis, liver failure, cirrhosis, carcinoma.
	1-5 y: 82-139%	
	6-17 y: 90-131%	
	>18 y: 80-120%	
Platelet aggregation	Results vary according to laboratory.	Collect 4-5 mL sample in sodium citrate tubes for analysis with light transmission aggregometer. Must be processed within 60 minutes of collection. Test measures the ability of platelets to aggregate and form clots in response to various activators. Decreased: Myeloproliferative disorders, autoimmune disorders, uremia, clotting disorders, and adverse effects of medications. Drugs that affect clotting should be avoided before test for up to 2 weeks (on advice of physician).

MIXING STUDIES AND FACTOR TESTING

Mixing studies are used to determine if abnormal test results for the PT and/or aPTT are because of coagulation deficiency or because of factor inhibitors. Because normal results still occur when PT and aPTT levels are at 50%, the test involves mixing equal amounts of the patient's plasma with a sample of plasma in which the coagulation factors are normal (leading to a 50% level). If the abnormal findings resulted from deficiency, the PT and aPTT results will be within normal range, but if the abnormal findings resulted from inhibitors, then the clotting times will be prolonged.

Factor testing is usually done when the PT and aPTT are abnormally prolonged (or in some cases for thrombosis) to determine the presence and type of clotting abnormality. Factor levels vary, so factor testing generally reports factors as a percentage of normal (which is 100%). Low percentages indicate hypocoagulopathy and percentages above 100% indicate hypercoagulopathy.

TYPES OF HEMOPHILIA

Hemophilia A is also referred to as "classic hemophilia". This is the most common form of hemophilia, and it is due to a deficiency in Factor VIII. Females are carriers. This disease affects males and leads to a prolonged clotting time and bleeding episodes. Less than 10 IU of factor VIII is characteristic of hemophilia A. Hemophilia A is 7 times more prevalent than Hemophilia B (Christmas disease), a deficiency or mutation of Factor IX. Christmas disease is also X-linked, and affects mostly males. People with Hemophilia B are at increased risk of hemorrhage. Finally, Hemophilia C is identified by the deficiency of Factor XI. This disease affects both sexes, and is an autosomal recessive disorder affecting primarily Jews of Ashkenazi descent. People with Hemophilia C often do not require treatment, and the disease is usually not severe. There is also no bleeding at the joints, as seen with Hemophilia A and B.

BERNARD-SOULIER SYNDROME

Bernard-Soulier syndrome is a disease that is due to the lack of glycoprotein Ib, which is normally present in the membranes of platelets. Glycoprotein Ib is the protein that reacts with the von Willebrand factor, and its absence causes problems in platelet aggregation and in the forming of blood clots. Platelets in a person with Bernard-Soulier syndrome are larger and more spherical than normal platelets, and their membranes are not as strong. This disease is inherited, and affects both males and females with an equal frequency.

CHRISTMAS DISEASE

Christmas disease is an inherited, X-chromosome linked disease affecting only males (because of their XY phenotype). Females are carriers. Christmas disease is characterized by the lack of clotting Factor IX, a protein that is normally found in plasma, necessary for platelet aggregation and the formation of blood clots. Without Factor IX, a patient is more likely to experience hemorrhage when injured, and abnormal bleeding episodes like nosebleeds, bruising, joint swelling, hematuria, hematochezia and melena. Christmas disease is sometimes called Hemophilia B. It is treated with regular injections of Factor IX. Classical Hemophilia A is treated with Factor VIII.

VON WILLEBRAND'S DISEASE

Von Willebrand's disease is a hereditary defect on Chromosome 12 that causes the von Willebrand factor, necessary for clotting, to either be absent or defective. Unlike Hemophilia A and B, both females and males can have von Willebrand's disease, and it especially targets people with blood type O. The von Willebrand factor (vWF) is a protein that aids in platelet aggregation and blood clotting, and it helps control platelet activity. Without the von Willebrand factor, or with a deficient factor, patients have menorraghia (heavy menstruation), epistaxis (nosebleeds), and bruising. Type I and II cases of von Willebrand's disease are mild and require no treatment, except when patients are undergoing surgery or dental work. Type III is severe, with spontaneous bleeding into their joints. Patients use Demoprexin, Cyklokapron, Amicar, and thrombin powder on cuts to control bleeding.

Immunology and Serology

IMMUNOGLOBULIN

An immunoglobulin is a glycoprotein that functions as an antibody. Immunoglobulins are produced by plasma cells. They function as antibodies by bonding with specific antigens. They play a huge role in the body's immune system. Immunoglobulins each contain four polypeptide chains. Two of them are deemed heavy (H), and two are light (L). There are five main classes of immunoglobulins. They are IgA, IgD, IgE, IgG, and IgM. Each of these classes is distinguished based on the type of heavy chains that they contain. IgA immunoglobulins contain alpha heavy chains. IgD immunoglobulins contain delta heavy chains, and IgE immunoglobulins contain epsilon heavy chains. IgG immunoglobulins contain gamma heavy chains, and IgM immunoglobulins contain mu heavy chains.

IMMUNOLOGY AND SEROLOGY TERMINOLOGY

Thermostable	Unaffected by heat.
Thermolabile	Easily affected by heat.
Physiologic(al)	Related to body functions.
Inactivation	Destruction of biological activity, such as by heat or other agent.
Complement	A group of blood proteins that go through a cascade of interactions as part of immune response.
Reagin	Complement-fixing antibody, IgE immunoglobulin that attaches to tissue cells in the species it derives from and interacts with antigen to cause release of histamine and other vasoactive amines.
Amboceptor	Old term for hemolysin.
Hemolysin	Antibody that binds to red blood cells and lyses them to release hemoglobin.
Cardiolipin	Phospholipid that increases with some disorders, such as autoimmune and coagulation disorders.
Monoclonal	Referring to a single clone; derived from a single cell.
Polyclonal	Referring to multiple clones; derived from multiple cells.

IMMUNOGLOBULINS IgA, IgD, AND IgE

IgA, IgD, and IgE are three of the five major classes of immunoglobulins. IgA immunoglobulins are found in various body secretions, such as tears, sweat, and saliva. They are also found in the respiratory and gastrointestinal tracts, where they serve as the main antibodies in these systems. The main function of IgA antibodies is to help protect the body against antigens that are ingested. They also help prevent any bacteria or viruses from attaching themselves to the skin and mucous membranes. IgD antibodies, on the other hand, are only found on B cells (lymphocytes). Their function has not been clearly defined. IgE antibodies are the antibodies that play a part in allergic reactions. They are created in the lungs, mucous membranes, and on the skin. This type of antibody is the least common.

IMMUNOGLOBULINS IgG AND IgM

IgG is the most common class of immunoglobulin. It is also the most abundant immunoglobulin class found in blood serum and in the lymphatic system. IgG helps protect the body against a variety of detrimental agents, such as viruses, bacteria, fungi, and foreign bodies. IgM antibodies are found in the various fluids of the body. They help stimulate the production of the IgG antibodies, and IgM antibodies are some of the first antibodies that are activated to respond to antigens in the body. These antibodies play a large role in the immune response to infections in the blood.

CROSS MATCHING

Cross matching is a test to determine if a unit of donated blood will be compatible with the blood of the intended recipient. There are two types of cross matching, major and minor. Major cross matching uses red blood cells from the donor's blood and the serum of the recipient to detect ABO compatibility or incompatibility, and to determine if the recipient's blood serum contains an antibody that will act against an antigen on the donor's red blood cells. Minor cross matching uses the red blood cells of the recipient and the blood serum from the donor. Minor cross matching can also detect ABO compatibility or incompatibility. It determines if the donor's plasma contains any antibodies that may act against antigens present on the surfaces of the red blood cells of the recipient. Minor cross matching is not used frequently.

PRINCIPLES OF IMMUNOLOGY

Immunology involves the immune response to foreign substances (microorganisms and proteins), which provides defense (attacks antigens/pathogens), homeostasis (digests damaged cellular materials), and surveillance (destroys mutated forms). All cells carry antigens, which are composed of proteins. The body usually recognizes its own antigens and does not attack them (except in autoimmune disorders). B-lymphocytes (produced in bone marrow) produce antigen-binding proteins (immunoglobulins) on their cell membranes. When the Ig binds with an antigen, this stimulates the B-cell to produce plasma cells, which in turn produce further immunoglobulins that are released as antibodies: IgM (first released), IgG (second released and more specific to an antigen), IgA (present in secretions) and IgE (triggers basophils and mast cells to release histamine). T-lymphocyte helper cells (CD4 cells) (produced in the thymus gland) secrete cytokines (hormones that signal other cells) when they contact foreign antigens. T-lymphocyte cytotoxic cells (CD8 cells) directly destroy foreign antigens that are outside of infected cells (not adhered).

FACTORS AFFECTING ANTIGEN-ANTIBODY REACTIONS

Factors affecting antigen-antibody reactions include:

- Temperature: Antigen-antibody reactions are usually more stable at low temperatures, and the strength of bonds tends to increase as the temperature rises.
- pH: Equilibrium constant is attained at 6.5-8.4. Extremes alter the antibody molecule.
- Incubation time: Duration needed to reach equilibrium varies according to the ionic strength: faster at low strength and slower at high strength. Duration should be at least 20 minutes at low strength.
- Ionic strength: Reactions vary in time needed to reach equilibrium depending on the concentration of ions. At low strength, gamma globulins aggregate, resulting in increased complement fraction attachment and RBV aggregation.
- Antibody/antigen excess: Numbers of antigens or antibodies are so high that antigen-antibody crosslinking (agglutination) is reduced because of the excess of either antigens or antibodies.
- Enhancement media: Reaction may vary depending on the type of enhancement media utilized.
- Blood-banking technology: Rare blood types may cause unexpected reactions.
- Dilution/Concentration: Can alter the number of immunoglobulins by increasing or decreasing dissociation.

GENERAL CHEMICAL STRUCTURE OF IMMUNOGLOBULINS

Immunoglobulins (antibodies) are glycoproteins. Glycoproteins are protein molecules that are attached to carbohydrate. Each immunoglobulin contains 4 polypeptide chains. Two of these chains are called heavy chains (H), which are further divided into alpha, delta, epsilon, gamma, and mu heavy chains. The other two chains are called light chains (L), and are further divided into kappa and lambda. The chains are all connected by disulfide bonds. The alpha chains are associated with IgA antibodies, delta chains with IgD antibodies, epsilon chains with IgE antibodies, gamma chains with IgG antibodies, and mu chains with IgM antibodies. Each chain present (heavy and light chains) also has two specific regions. These regions are called the amino-terminal variable region (V) and the carboxyl-terminal variable region (C). There is a lot of variability in the V regions in the different antibody classes, however, there is not a lot of variability in the C regions.

HLA SYSTEM

HLA stands for human leukocyte antigen. The human leukocyte antigens are part of the major histocompatibility complex (MHC), a region found on chromosome 6. HLAs are found in all nucleated cells in the body. HLAs are inherited from one's parents and are practically unique to a particular individual. There are four main types of human leukocyte antigens, HLA-A, HLA-B, HLA-C, and HLA-D. Human leukocyte antigens help encode proteins on the surfaces of nucleated cells, and they play an important role in helping the body distinguish its own cells from foreign cells. Therefore, HLAs are very important when it comes to human organ transplant rejection or acceptance. In the laboratory, HLA-A, HLA-B, and HLA-C antigens can be identified using blood serum, however, HLA-D antigens can only be identified by the use of a mixed lymphocyte culture.

KELL BLOOD GROUP SYSTEM

The Kell blood group system is composed of four antigens that are found in red blood cells (erythrocytes). These four antigens are K (Kell), k (Cellano), Kpa, and Kpb. The particular phenotype known as the knull phenotype (K-k-Kp(a-b-)) has been implicated in chronic granulomatous disease (CGD). In this disease, neutrophils cannot produce hydrogen peroxide to kill invading bacteria and viruses. The antibodies to the Kell antigens are the IgG antibodies, and IgG antibodies can play a part in hemolytic disease of the newborn, as well as in adverse patient reactions to transfusions.

DUFFY BLOOD GROUP SYSTEM

The Duffy blood group system is a group of antigens (proteins) found on the outsides of erythrocytes (red blood cells). They are distinguished based on their reactions with anti-Fyᵃ serum. Blood can be said to be Duffy positive, meaning that the Duffy antigen is present on the red blood cells. Blood can also be said to be Duffy negative, meaning that there is no Duffy antigen present. There are three common Duffy phenotypes, and they are Fy(a⁺b⁺), Fy(a⁺b⁻), and Fy(a⁻b⁺). Almost all whites are Duffy positive, and almost all blacks of African descent are Duffy negative. Because the Duffy antigen is a receptor for the parasites that can cause malaria, being Duffy negative (not having the Duffy antigen) can help provide resistance against contracting malaria. Furthermore, if a person who is Duffy negative receives blood that is Duffy positive in a blood transfusion, an allergic reaction can occur.

IMPLICATION OF THE RHESUS FACTOR IN RHESUS DISEASE OF THE NEWBORN

In Rhesus disease of the newborn, a pregnant woman who is Rh D negative is pregnant with a baby who is Rh D positive. A tiny quantity of the fetus' Rh D positive blood enters the mother's blood stream. The mother, in turn, creates antibodies against the Rh D antigen in the fetus' blood. These antibodies can then pass back through the placenta to the fetus, and if there are enough antibodies present, they destroy the fetus's red blood cells. The destruction of these red blood cells is called Rhesus disease of the newborn or hemolytic disease of the newborn. A woman's first pregnancy may seem unaffected, but she can be sensitized during it. The disease gets worse with subsequent pregnancies as antibodies increase, unless RhoGAM injections are given preventatively during pregnancy and after delivery.

ANTIBODIES ASSOCIATED WITH VARIOUS CONDITIONS

1. Cold agglutination syndrome is most often associated with IgM antibodies.
2. Paroxysmal cold hemoglobinuria is most often associated with IgG antibodies.
3. Warm autoimmune hemolytic anemia is most often associated with IgG antibodies. Sometimes, IgA antibodies can play a part in this form of anemia.
4. Hemolytic disease of the newborn is most often associated with IgG antibodies, primarily because they are the only antibodies that can cross the placenta from the mother to the fetus.

SYPHILIS

Syphilis is a bacterial infection caused by the spirochete *Treponema pallidum* and transmitted through oral, anal, or vaginal sex and needle sharing. The incubation period is 10 to 90 days. There are 3 stages to the disease:

- Primary (3-8 weeks): Chancre (painless) in areas of sexual contact, very contagious.
- Secondary (1-2 years): General flu-like symptoms (sore throat, fever, headaches) and red papular rash on trunk, flexor surfaces, palms, and soles, hair loss, and lymphadenopathy occur about 3-6 weeks after end of primary phase and eventually resolves.
- Tertiary/Late (latent >2 years): Affects about 30% and includes CNS (psychoses, confusion, ataxia, aphasia) and cardiovascular symptoms 3-20 years after initial infection. Gummas (granulomatous lesions) may be widespread. Complications include dementia, meningitis, neuropathy, and thoracic aneurysm. Noncontagious after 4 years.

Women who are infected may transmit the disease to a fetus, resulting in congenital syphilis. The infant may be born with no obvious symptoms at birth or may be born with physical changes associated with advanced syphilis.

BRUTON'S DISEASE

Bruton's disease is a condition in which there is a deficiency of all 5 major classes of immunoglobulins. This disease is sometimes referred to as agammaglobulinemia. It is a recessive, X-linked disorder that affects only males. A patient with Bruton's disease does not produce B-lymphocytes. Patients will have recurrent pneumonia and sinusitis, poor growth, bowel disease, encephalitis, and may die by age 40. Bruton's disease can be detected by amniocentesis. Patients who get IgG injections by age 5 have less morbidity and mortality. In the laboratory, serum levels of IgA, IgD, IgE, and IgM antibodies may not be detected, and IgG antibodies may also be absent or barely detectable. However, the lack of a gamma globulin peak during serum electrophoresis can indicate the existence of Bruton's disease.

DIRECT COOMBS TEST

The direct Coombs test is used to determine if complement system factors or antibodies are bound to antigens found on the surface of red blood cells in a test sample. In this test, a patient's test sample is washed, which removes the serum from the red blood cells. The red blood cells are then added to the Coombs reagent. The Coombs reagent is an antihuman globulin. The antihuman globulin will cause the red blood cells in the test sample to clot (agglutinate) if those red blood cells have antibodies or complement system factors attached to their surfaces. This result is indicative of a positive direct Coombs test. If the agglutination does not occur, then the direct Coombs test is negative. The direct Coombs test is used most often if hemolytic anemia (immune controlled) is suspected. In patients whose red blood cells are being hemolyzed by their immune system, a positive Coombs test will occur.

INDIRECT COOMBS TEST

The indirect Coombs test is performed in vitro to understand and determine the presence of reactions between antibodies and antigens in a red blood cell sample. In the laboratory, red blood cells are washed and then added to a test serum. If the test serum contains red blood cells that have antigens or antibodies attached to their surfaces, the antibodies will bind onto the surfaces of the washed red blood cells. Next, the red blood cells are then washed several more times with a saline solution, and then added to the Coombs reagent (an antihuman globulin). If antibodies attached to the washed red blood cells previously, the red blood cells will clot (agglutinate) when the Coombs reagent is added. If the agglutination occurs, the indirect Coombs test positive. The indirect Coombs test can be used for: Antibody identification, determining antibody concentrations in serum or plasma before blood transfusion, titrations, or determining red blood cell phenotypes.

KLEIHAUER-BETKE TEST

The Kleihauer-Betke test is an acid elution test used to determine the severity or presence of fetal-maternal hemorrhage postpartum. This is accomplished by determining the quantity of fetal red blood cells or hemoglobin present in the mother's blood stream after delivery. This test is performed when a Rh negative mother has given birth. In this particular test, at a pH of 3.2, a sample of maternal blood is stained with erythrosine B-hematoxylin. Once the stain is applied, the adult hemoglobin (which is soluble in the acid solution) will turn pale. Sometimes the adult hemoglobin is said to become ghost-like. The fetal hemoglobin, on the other end, is not soluble in the acid solution, and remains bright pink. Depending on the amount of fetal hemoglobin present in the maternal blood sample, the appropriate dosage of Rh immune globulin (RhIg) can be administered to the mother to help prevent the formation of Rh antibodies in the mother's blood.

WEIL-FELIX TEST

The Weil-Felix test is used to define the presence of *Rickettsia*, bacteria that are often carried by lice, ticks, and fleas. Populations of *Rickettsia* that are present in an affected patient's blood serum cause the production of various antibodies. These antibodies have the ability to react with other types of bacteria. In the Weil-Felix test, another type of bacteria (often *Proteus vulgaris*) is added to a patient's blood serum. This bacteria serves as an antigen and will react (agglutinate) with the antibodies produced from the *Rickettsia* in the patient's blood serum. This agglutination can help identify which type of *Rickettsia* afflicts the patient. Some rickettsial diseases that can be identified by this method are Rocky Mountain spotted fever, trench fever, typhus, and scrub typhus.

ELISA TEST

ELISA stands for enzyme-linked immunosorbent assay, an immunoassay test that identifies the presence of specific substances, like the AIDS virus. ELISA can identify hormones, proteins, antibodies, or antigens. Add an antibody specific to the substance of interest to the test system. Mix a sample of the pure substance in question with an enzyme. This creates an enzyme-linked substance. Add both the enzyme-linked substance and the blood serum to the test system. If the serum contains the substance of interest, less of the enzyme-linked substance will be able to bind to the antibody that was added. If there is no substance of interest in the serum, more enzyme-linked substance will be able to bond to the available antibody. Finally, add the particular substance that the enzyme acts on to the system. Measure the product produced via a color analysis. This test is very sensitive and is used frequently to confirm a less sensitive, but cheaper, screening test.

MICROHEMAGGLUTINATION TEST FOR TREPONEMA PALLIDUM (MHA-TP)

The **microhemagglutination test for *Treponema pallidum* (MHA-TP),** a gram-negative spirochete, is a nontreponemal antibody tests that assesses serum for antibodies to syphilis although this particular test has been generally replaced by other tests that are more specific, such as fluorescent treponemal antibody absorption (FTA-ABS), immunoassays, and molecular testing. MHA-TP can be used to confirm a positive diagnosis of syphilis on other tests. MHA-TP is able to detect antibodies to *T. pallidum* and is used for all stages of syphilis except during the first month of infection. One of the problems with MHA-TP is that false positives may occur in the presence of other infections, so it is not specific to syphilis: mononucleosis, Lyme disease, malaria, relapsing fever, leptospirosis, and leprosy. Patients with systemic lupus erythematosus may also have a false-positive on the test.

FEBRILE AGGLUTINATION TESTS

Febrile agglutinins are antibodies that are active at normal body temperature and can cause their antigens (such as RBCs, proteins) to clump when exposed to each other, resulting in a fever. Febrile agglutinins are present in some disorders, such as systemic lupus erythematosus, hemolytic anemia, inflammatory bowel disease, and lymphoma. They may also occur in response to some infections (salmonella, brucellosis, typhoid fever) and when taking some medications (penicillin, methyldopa), so these medications may interfere with test results. To identify an infection, a blood sample is taken when a patient is actively infected (with fever and symptoms) or during convalescence, diluted (20-40 times), and mixed with antigens of a specific infectious microorganism. This sample is then examined to determine if an antigen-antibody reaction has occurred. Increased IgM usually indicates a new infection and increased IgG indicates a chronic infection or history of infection.

C-REACTIVE PROTEIN AGGLUTINATION SLIDE TESTS

C-reactive protein (CRP) agglutination slide tests can be used to screen patients for CRP (qualitative test) or to determine the titer (quantitative test). A number of different test kits are available, so procedures may vary.

Qualitative test	Quantitative test
Add latex solution to positive and negative controls and serum (or diluted and undiluted serum), mix, and agitate for 2 minutes to observe for agglutination (clumping) in serum, a reaction indicating the presence of C-reactive protein.	Mix serum samples to different dilutions in saline and conduct test similar to qualitative method to determine the highest dilution that shows agglutination (positive reaction).

ANTISTREPTOLYSIN SCREEN AND TITER

Antistreptolysin O screen and titer (ASO) identifies the presence of streptolysin O antibodies, which form in response to the streptolysin O enzyme (antigen) secreted by group A β-hemolytic streptococci. The antibodies are present within one week and peak at 2-3 weeks after onset of streptococcal infection. Increased titer is present with strep-associated rheumatic fever, scarlet fever, endocarditis, and glomerulonephritis.

RHEUMATOID ARTHRITIS (RA) TESTS

Rheumatoid factor (RF)	Normal value 0-20 IU/mL.
	Assesses for macroglobulin type antibody that is present in connective tissue disease. Non-specific for RA
Anti-citrullinated protein antibody (ACPA):	Normal values: Negative: <20. Weakly positive: 20-39. Moderately positive: 40-59. Strongly positive: >60.
	Assesses for autoantibodies against citrullinated proteins, to which those with RA react.
Erythrocyte sedimentation rate (ESR):	Normal values: Age <50: 0-15 mm/h males and 0-25 mm/h females. Age >50: 0-20 mm/h males and 0-30 mm/h females.
	Inflammation causes increased globulins or fibrinogens, and these cause RBCs to clump and fall to the bottom of a vertical test tube. ESR is nonspecific for RA, but increased ESR may indicate increased inflammation.
C-reactive protein (CRP):	Normal value <1 mg/dL.
	Assesses for abnormal glycoproteins, which are produced by the liver when inflammation is present. CRP is non-specific for RA.

SYSTEMATIC LUPUS ERYTHEMATOSUS (SLE OR LE) TESTS

Systemic lupus erythematosus (SLE) is a chronic connective tissue disorder believed triggered by an antibody-antigen immune response to an environmental agent, resulting in widespread damage of vessels and organs, primarily in females. SLE ranges from mild to widely disseminated, and may include arthralgia, "butterfly" rash, arthritis, anemia, leukopenia, visceral lesions, CNS involvement (seizures, headaches, psychosis), fever, and lymphadenopathy. There is no single specific test for SLE, but rather diagnosis is based on the results of a number of imaging studies (x-rays, ECG) and laboratory studies:

- Complete blood cell count (CDC): May show anemia with erythrocytopenia and/or leukopenia.
- Erythrocyte sedimentation rate (ESR): Rate increases with SLE.
- Renal and hepatic function tests: Abnormalities may indicate lesions in the kidneys or liver.
- Urinalysis: Protein may be in the urine with renal lesions.
- Antinuclear antibody test: Presence of antibodies indicates an immune response. While results are not specific to ANA, this test is used primarily as part of SLE diagnosis.
- Renal biopsy: To determine type and degree of kidney involvement.

ANTINUCLEAR ANTIBODY (ANA) TESTS

ANA is used to diagnose autoimmune disorders, primarily SLE, Sjögren syndrome, scleroderma, and rheumatic diseases, which involve multiple body systems. Diagnosis depends on the ANA pattern exhibited and associated antibodies. Laboratories vary in reference ranges. Antinuclear antibodies are autoimmune antibodies that mistakenly target native tissue and cells as foreign. ANA is often done in conjunction with other autoantibody tests, such as anti-DNA and anti-nucleolar.

Results	Testing
Positive or negative: ANA results vary depending on the specific test used and the lab.	Collect serum (3 mL) in red-capped tube for indirect fluorescent antibody (IFA) or immunoassay. Immunoassay is less sensitive that IFA, so initial screening may be done by immunoassay with confirmation testing by IFA.

ANTIGEN DETECTION

Antigen detection for specific organisms is frequently done as part of diagnostic studies. Various tests can be used. Enzyme immunoassays (EIA/ELISA) use various techniques, depending on the target antigen and microorganism. Techniques include binding an antibody (specific to the antigen under study) to a micro-dilution tray and adding the antigen, incubating, and washing it. Then, a second enzyme-labeled antibody is utilized to detect the antigen through a color change. With use of the immunochromatographic membrane, an antigen is absorbed through a nitrocellulose membrane and the color change occurs on the membrane when reagents are added. Latex agglutination tests, in which the antigen is affixed to latex beads, are used to identify carbohydrate antigens that occur on encapsulated organisms. With the Western blot test, antigens are put on a nitrocellulose strip and incubated with the antibody specimen and treated with an enzyme-labeled antibody and color change observed. Western blot is used frequently to confirm diagnosis of HIV.

PREGNANCY TESTS

Human chorionic gonadotropin (hCG) (quantitative)	Negative: <5 mIU/mL	Measures the amount of hCG in the blood.
	2 weeks: 5-100 mIU/mL	
	4 weeks: 10,000-80,000 mIU/mL	
	5-12 weeks: 90,000-500,000 mIU/mL	Obtain 1 mL sample in red or tiger-capped tube or 1 mL in heparinized green-capped tube for immunoassay.
	13-24 weeks: 5000-80,000 mIU/mL	
	26-28 weeks: 3000-15,000 mIU/mL	
hCG (qualitative)	Negative if absent	Measures only presence or absence of hCG and cannot determine weeks of gestation.
	Positive if present	Obtain 1 mL sample in red or tiger-capped tube or 1 mL in heparinized green-capped tube.
hCG urine (home-pregnancy test)	Positive or negative	A test strip of some type is used and color change noted.

VIRAL/RETROVIRAL LABORATORY TESTS

Cytomegalovirus	Negative: ≤0.9 index	Obtain 1 mL sample in red-capped tube for enzyme immunoassay for antibody detection.
	Indeterm: 0.91-1.09	
	Positive: ≥1.1 index	
Retrovirus	Negative: 0 present	Obtain 1 mL sample in red or tiger-capped tube for enzyme immunoassay for antibody detection. Tests may include ELISA, nucleic acid testing, PCR, western blot.
Epstein-Barr	Negative <17 u/mL	Obtain 1 mL sample in gold-capped serum separator tube for chemiluminescent immunoassay.
	Indeterm 18.0-21.9 u/mL	
	Positive >22 u/mL	
Rubella	Negative: ≤0.9 index	Obtain 1 mL sample in red-capped tube for chemiluminescent immunoassay.
	Indeterm: 0.91-1.09	
	Positive: ≥1.1 index	

ANTI-HUMAN IMMUNODEFICIENCY VIRUS (HIV) TESTS

These tests screen for the presence of antibodies and/or antigens to HIV. The antigen is present before antibodies, so tests that include antigen assessment can give earlier results.

Rapid HIV test	Negative or positive	Most test only for antibodies, but newer tests may test for antigens as well. Tests can be done on blood, plasma, or oral fluid, but the rapid test is most often done with an oral swab with results (usually color change) available within seconds to minutes, depending on the test. These tests are less accurate than other tests, so findings must be confirmed.
HIV-1/HIV-2 test (serum)	Negative or positive	Screens for HIV antigen (p24) and HIV-1 and HIV-2 antibodies. Obtain 1 mL sample in red-capped tube for enzyme immunoassay. Confirmatory tests required.
IFA/Western blot	Negative or positive	Done for confirmatory testing when initial screening tests are positive or with individuals at high risk with negative screening tests.

Immunohematology

Antihuman globulin (Coombs)	Animal (commonly rabbit) serum immunized with human globulin that has been purified to prepare antibodies against immunoglobulin G (IgG) and complement.
Direct antihuman globulin test	RBCs washed to remove serum and unbound antibodies and the antihuman globulin added. Agglutination occurs with presence of antibody. Test used to detect sensitized RBCs in erythroblastosis fetalis and autoimmune hemolytic anemia.
Indirect antihuman globulin test	Serum incubated with donor RBCs, cells washed, and antiglobulin added. If cells absorb antibody, agglutination occurs: Used for blood typing and adverse transfusion reactions.
Compatibility testing	Testing carried out between the patient's blood specimen and the donor's blood specimen to ensure the blood types are compatible. Includes blood typing of patient and donor, repeat donor testing, forward, reverse, and weak D (Du) cross match testing and further testing as indicated for discrepancies.
Auto control/Autoimmunity	Condition in which a humoral or cell-mediated response to components of body tissue (autoantigens) results in hypersensitivity reactions or autoimmune disease in which antibodies attack the body'

IMMUNOGEN, ANTIGEN, HAPTEN, ADJUVANT, AND ANTIBODY

1. Immunogen: any substance that produces an immune response
2. Antigen: any substance that reacts with substances in the immune system; antigens do not always produce an immune response
3. Hapten: a molecule with a low molecular weight, which combines with another molecule to produce an antibody response
4. Adjuvant: a substance that magnifies immune responses
5. Antibody: a protein that fixes itself to an antigen; also known as immunoglobulins, and divided into five classes: IgA, IgD, IgE, IgG, and IgM

POLYCLONAL HYPERGAMMAGLOBULINEMIA AND MONOCLONAL HYPERGAMMAGLOBULINEMIA

1. Polyclonal hypergammaglobulinemia: a broad spike in the gamma region of the protein electrophoresis performed on a serum; indicates elevated levels of specific antibodies; the result of infectious disease, liver disease, or inflammation
2. Monoclonal hypergammaglobulinemia: a narrow peak in the gamma region of a protein electrophoresis performed on a serum; due to malignant transformation of a B lymphocyte clone; the results of multiple myeloma, immunoglobulin heavy chain diseases, or Waldenström's macroglobulinemia

TERMS RELATED TO TRANSPLANT IMMUNOLOGY

1. Allograft: tissue is transplanted from one place to another on the same individual
2. Isograft: tissue from one individual is transplanted onto a genetically identical individual

109

3. Autograft: tissue from one individual is transplanted onto an individual from the same species
4. Graft acceptance: the condition in which healing and revascularization signal the acceptance of a tissue graft or transplant
5. Hyperacute graft rejection: rejection of a graft or transplant in the first 24 hours
6. Acute graft rejection: rejection of a graft or transplant within weeks
7. Chronic graft rejection: rejection of a graft or transplant within months or years

ANTIBODY-ANTIGEN REACTIONS IN THE LABORATORY

1. Labeled immunoassay: a test in which a label, like enzyme, radionucleotide, fluorochrome, or chemiluminescent molecule, is affixed to an antibody or antigen so that results may be measured
2. Agglutination reaction: Lab test in which a soluble antigen reacts to a soluble antibody or vice versa; examples may be reactions between different ABO blood types or the hCG agglutination reaction
3. Precipitation reaction: laboratory tests in which soluble anti-bodies react with soluble antigens, as for instance the tests radial immunodiffusion, double gel diffusion, immunofixation, immunoelectrophoresis, nephelometry, and turbidimetry

BLOOD TYPING

ABO system: The H (O) antigen, located on chromosome 19, is a precursor to ABO antigens and is found in all people except those with the Bombay Blood type. Type O blood has only this antigen attached to the surface of erythrocytes while type A, B and AB carry one or two additional antigens with phenotype based on the presence or absence of A and/or B antigens. Type O lacks both. In the ABO system, agglutinins (antibodies) to A and/or B are also present. Type A has the anti-B antibody; type B, the anti-A; type AB, neither anti-A nor anti-B; and type O, both anti-A and anti-B. Type O ("universal recipient") may develop a mild reaction to A or B blood because of the presence of these antibodies. Structure:

- H/O antigen: Fucose—2 galactose—N-acetylglucosamine—glucose
- A antigen: Fucose—2 galactose—N-acetylglucosamine—glucose—N-acetylgalactosamine
- B antigen: Fucose—3 galactose—N-acetylglucosamine—glucose

When antibodies encounter foreign antigens on erythrocytes, antibodies bind to the antigens and cause the blood cells to begin to agglutinate (clump) and hemolyze.

ABO blood typing:

- Forward: Reagent that contains anti-A and anti-B antibodies used to determine presence or absence of A and/or B antigens on surface of erythrocytes.
- Reverse: Reagent that contains A1 and B antigen used to test serum for anti-A and/or anti-B antibodies to confirm forward testing. Any discrepancy must be resolved before blood transfusion. For example, the patient may have the A2 subgroup and may require additional testing to identify that subgroup.
- D (Rh): Rh+ individuals carry the D antigen and Rh- do not, but the anti-D antibody is not naturally occurring but occurs as part of the immune response when Rh- blood comes in contact with Rh+ blood, such as may occur during pregnancy when Rh+ fetal cells pass into maternal circulation or from a transfusion. Erythrocytes are tested with a reagent with anti-D antibody.

- Du (weak D): Because some D+ cells have a weak antigen and do not react to anti-D antibodies, further testing for the weak D is carried out with the cells incubated, washed and anti-human globulin added to determine if agglutination (weak D positive) occurs.

RBC ANTIGEN PHENOTYPING AND FREQUENCY OF ANTIGEN DISTRIBUTION

Erythrocyte (RBC) phenotyping is done based on the type of antigen on the cell surface with A, B, AB, and O the 4 primary phenotypes, but there are many other antigens present, and these antigens are not usually tested for with blood typing although it may be necessary for some patients, especially if discrepancies occur with typing or patients have known subtypes or rare blood types (RzR, Jk [a-b], Di [b], Dr [a-]). Antigen distribution (average, USA):

O—Rh+: 39%	A—Rh-: 6%
A—Rh+: 31%	AB—Rh+: 3%
B—RH+: 9%	B—Rh-: 2%
O—RH-: 9%	AB—Rh-: 1%

Distribution varies according to ethnicity and matching may be easier within the same ethnic group. For example, while 39% of people are O—Rh+, this ranges from 37% of Caucasians, 39% Asians, 47% African Americans, to 53% Asians. Indigenous populations in South and Central America are almost 100% type O—Rh+.

ANTIBODY IDENTIFICATION TESTS

Phases of reactivity, phases involved in reacting donor RBCs with recipient's serum for compatibility testing, include:

- Saline phase: Donor RBCs are suspended in saline and combined at room temperature with the serum (which contains the recipient's antibodies) to determine if an antigen-antibody reaction (agglutination) occurs. This phase recognizes ABO incompatibility. "Immediate spin" variation includes only centrifugation and examination (no incubation) and takes 5 minutes. Hemolysis during this phase indicates the presence of cold agglutinins. Antibodies that react are usually IgM.
- Thermophase with protein phase: RBCs suspended in the antibody serum are incubated for 30 minutes at 37°C with 22% albumin OR with low ionic strength saline (LISS) to enhance agglutination of univalent antibodies, such as Rh (D). LISS requires 15 minutes incubation time. (This phase of testing may be omitted if testing with antihuman globulin is conducted.) Antibodies that react are usually IgM or IgG.
- Antihuman globulin (Coombs) phase: Cells are washed and react with AHG reagent, indicating antibody sensitivity. Antibodies that react are usually IgG.

Enhancement media are those used to increase detection of antibodies. Commonly used enhancement media include albumin and low ionic strength solution. (LISS). Polyethylene glycol (PEG) and albumin (22%) may be used together as enhancement media for the direct antihuman globulin (Coombs) test) to aid in differentiating significant from insignificant antibodies as the enhancement media reduces the time needed for incubation as well as promoting agglutination and reducing zeta potential. Both PEG and albumin enhance agglutination, and PEG enhances antibody uptake but can also cause red blood cell aggregation if centrifuged. Enzymes, such as papain and ficin, may also be used to enhance antibody detection.

Rule-out is a procedure used in an antibody screen to determine if antigens are reacting to antibodies. Each cell is assessed as to whether or not it reacted to various antibodies. For example,

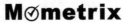

if the screen shows no reaction between an antigen and the anti-Fy^a antibody, then this antibody is ruled out.

SCREENING FOR ANTIGEN NEGATIVE BLOOD IN A NORMAL POPULATION AND PROPERLY USING POSITIVE AND NEGATIVE CONTROLS

Antigen-negative blood: While blood typing for the normal population is done for ABO and RH (D) antigens, there are over 300 antigens on red blood cells (RBCs), and patients can develop antibodies to any of these antigens. In most cases the antibody-antigen reaction is so mild it is of no consequence, but severe reactions can occur. These reactions become evident during the thermophase and/or antihuman globulin phases of testing. These patients must receive blood that is antigen-negative for the antigens to which they have antibodies that may result in reaction. For antigens with a fairly high rate of frequency, screening may be done locally, but for more obscure antigens, screening may need to be done in reference laboratories with large numbers of controls available. Negative controls are used for positive presence of antigens, and positive controls for negative presence, and these must carefully match the RBCs or errors will occur.

ANTIGEN DISTRIBUTION AND PROVISION OF ANTIGEN-NEGATIVE BLOOD FOR TRANSFUSION

When a patient has antibodies to specific antigens and must receive antigen-negative blood for transfusion, a problem that most often occurs in patients who undergo more than 15 transfusions and develop antibodies to minor antigens, the number of units that must be tested depends upon the **antigen distribution**. For example, if an antigen is found in about 20% of a population, one can estimate that 20% of units of blood contain that specific antigen (even though the actual percentage may be higher or lower). If a patient must receive 2 units of blood, the formula to estimate the number that must be tested for compatibility is:

\# of units ordered/percentage of units containing the antigen

2/0.20 = 10 units

If the patient carries antibodies to more than 1 antigen and must receive blood that is antigen-negative for both types, then the calculations must take both into consideration.

BLOOD GROUP SYSTEMS AND ANTIGEN DISTRIBUTION

Rh (subtypes D, C, E, c, e)	Cause severe delayed hemolytic reactions with primarily IgG antibodies (some IgM present).
	D frequency: Whites—85%, Blacks—92%, Asians—99%
	C frequency: Whites—68%, Blacks—27%, Asians—93%
	E frequency: Whites—29%, Blacks—22%, Asians—39%
	c frequency: Whites—80%, Blacks—96%, Asians—47%
	e frequency: Whites—98%, Blacks—98%, Asians—96%
MNS blood types	Carried on glycophorins on RBC cell membrane. Hemolytic reactions are rare but may be severe, with Igg and IgM antibodies.
	M frequency: Whites—78%, Blacks—74%
	N frequency: Whites—72%, Blacks—75%
	S frequency: Whites—55%, Blacks—31%
	s frequency—Whites—89%, Blacks 93%

TESTS TO ELUTE ANTIBODIES FROM RED BLOOD CELLS

When the direct Coombs test is positive, the **heat elution procedure** is indicated. The antigen-antibody bond of cells coated with antigens is disrupted to free the antibodies, which are then collected in saline or 6% albumin solution for testing with reagent cells. Procedures may vary somewhat, depending on laboratory protocol. Heat elution:

- Wash 1 mL sensitized RBCs 5 times in normal saline to remove free antibodies.
- Wash again in a volume of saline equal to RBC volume and centrifuge at 1500 rpm for 60 seconds.
- Test supernatant for free antibodies and repeat last wash procedure until no antibodies are detected. The supernatant of the final wash serves as the negative control.
- Place volume of saline equal to RBC volume in centrifuge tube and incubate in 56°C water bath for 10 minutes.
- Centrifuge (prewarmed cups) at 3400 rpm for 69 seconds.
- Remove supernatant fluid (should be hemoglobin tinted), which serves as the elute.
- Test elute for presence of antibodies.

SALIVA TESTING

Saliva and other body fluids may contain a water-soluble blood group substance in about four-fifths of the population. These people are positive secretors. Substances secreted by blood type include: A (A and small amount H), B (B and small amount H), O (H), and AB (A, B, and small amount H). **Saliva testing for secretor status**:

Obtain 2-3 mL saliva sample.

- Place tube in water bath (boiling) for 10 minutes to inactivate enzymes.
- Cool for short period of time.
- Place in centrifuge tube and centrifuge for 4 minutes.
- Prepare 3 tubes and label: A, B, and H.
- Prepare 2 tubes and label: A, B, and H controls.
- Place 1 drop of diluted antiserum in each tube (anti-A in A test/control tubes, etc.)
- Place 1 drop of saliva in each test tube and 1 drop of saline in each control tube and mix.
- Incubate (room temperature) for 10 minutes.
- Place 1 drop reagent red cells in each test and control tube (A-1 for A, B for B, and screening cell I or II for H).
- Incubate again as above.
- Centrifuge as needed for saline reaction.
- Note agglutination. Control tubes should show agglutination and test tubes none if negative secretor status.

FLUID-PHASE PRECIPITATION REACTION

In a fluid-phase precipitation reaction, the antigen and antibody are soluble and tend toward diffusion. The reaction is accomplished as follows: a soluble antigen in solution is placed on top of a soluble antibody in solution, at which point the antigen and antibody diffuse into one another. A precipitate is formed, directly proportional to the concentrations of the antibody and antigen.

PRECIPITATION REACTIONS

1. Double immunodiffusion: soluble antibody and soluble antigen diffuse into agarose gel, with a line forming at the intersection of optimum concentrations of each; test is performed to identify a particular antibody, as well is to determine the concentration of that antibody in serum
2. Countercurrent immunoelectrophoresis: soluble antibody and soluble antigen are placed in separate wells on agarose gel plate; the addition of electric current stimulates the two substances to move towards one another, forming a line at their respective optimum concentrations; test is performed to determine the presence of antibodies to infectious agents, autoantibodies, and microbial agents
3. Immunofixation electrophoresis (IFE): sample of urine, serum, or cerebral spinal fluid is subjected to electrophoresis on an agarose gel plate, after which a cellulose acetate strip is placed on top; antibodies in the strip will diffuse into the gel, forming a precipitate; this test is performed to identify the presence of a specific antibody
4. The rocket technique: an antiserum which makes up part of the electrophoresis gel is combined with antigens in a sample subjected to electrophoresis; a rocket-shaped precipitate is formed

AGGLUTINATION REACTIONS VS. PRECIPITATION REACTIONS

- Agglutination reaction: use either soluble antibodies with solid antigens or solid antibodies with soluble antigens; provide semi-quantitative or qualitative results; examples include column agglutination and complement fixation
- Precipitation reaction: choose a soluble antigens and soluble antibodies; require more time than agglutination reactions; may have quantitative, semi-quantitative, or qualitative results; examples include radial immunodiffusion and turbidimetry

TYPES OF AGGLUTINATION REACTIONS

1. Direct agglutination: naturally occurring antigens are used
2. Viral agglutination: viruses agglutinate to red blood cells after viruses affix to surface receptors on red blood cells
3. Passive agglutination: specific soluble antigens attached or particles, resulting in agglutination, and indicating the presence of specific antigens
4. Reverse passive agglutination: specific antibodies attached to particles, indicating the presence of specific antigens

TYPES OF IMMUNOFLUORESCENCE REACTIONS

1. Direct immunofluorescence: reagent antibody labeled with fluorescent dye reacts to a specific antigen, forming an antigen-antibody complex, and thereby suggesting the existence of a particular antigen
2. Indirect immunofluorescence: unlabeled antibody reacts with antigens and a sample, forming an antigen-antibody complex; at this point, the antigen-antibody complex reacts with another labeled antibody, forming an antibody-antigen-antibody complex
3. Biotin-avidin immunofluorescence: a form of indirect immunofluorescence in which a labeled antibody and a labeled fluorochrome react with an antigen

CLASSES OF ANTIBODIES

Every antibody has two heavy polypeptide chains and two light polypeptide chains. The identity of the heavy chains depends on the class of antibody. The light chains will be either kappa or lambda chains. Each polypeptide chain has a variable region, which identifies the particular antibody, and one or more constant regions. All of the chains are joined by disulfide bonds.

BLOOD GROUP SYSTEMS AND ANTIGEN DISTRIBUTION

Fy (a, b, 3) (Duffy)	Common in those with malaria (*Plasmodium vivax*). Hemolytic reaction is usually mild to moderate delayed, with primarily IgG antibodies.
	Fy-a frequency: Whites—66%, Blacks—10%, Asians—99%.
	Fy-b frequency: Whites—83%, Blacks—23%, Asians—17.5%.
	Fy-3 frequency: Whites—100%, Blacks—32%, Asians—99%.
Jk (a, b, 3) (Kidd)	Cause delayed hemolytic reactions, with IgG and IgM antibodies (primarily IgG).
	Jk-a frequency: Whites—77%, Blacks—92%, Asians—73%. J
	k-b frequency: Whites—74%, Blacks—49%, Asians—23%.
	Jk-3 frequency: Whites, Blacks, and Asians—100%.

COLD AGGLUTININS

Cold agglutinins (cold-reacting) are autoantibodies (primarily IgM) that activate and cause red blood cell agglutination at cold temperatures (0° to 10°C). Cold agglutinins may cause severe hemolytic reactions during transfusions. Cold agglutinins are primarily associated with *Mycoplasma pneumoniae* infection, viral infections, and lymphoreticular cancers. Pathogenicity is dependent on the cold agglutinins' ability to bind to RBCs and to activate complement. Normal findings: Agglutination not evident with titers ≤1:16.

FEBRILE AGGLUTININS

Febrile agglutinins (warm-reacting) are autoantibodies (primarily IgG) that activate at normal body temperature. Febrile agglutinins are associated with lymphoma, leukemia, and a number of infectious diseases, include salmonellosis, brucellosis, tularemia, Rocky Mountain spotted fever, and murine typhus. Normal findings: Agglutination not evident at titers ≤1:80.

NATURALLY OCCURRING ANTIBODIES

Naturally occurring antibodies are those found in the body that were not produced in response to an antigen but through cross-reactivity or exposure to environmental agents with properties similar to antigen, such as dust and bacteria. Naturally occurring antibodies are usually IgM.

RED BLOOD CELLS FOR PATIENTS WITH SPECIAL NEEDS REQUIREMENTS

Cytomegalovirus (CMV) negative blood is from donors who have been tested for CMV IgG antibodies and found negative. These blood units (red blood cells and platelets) are labeled as CMV negative but this does not completely reduce the risk of transmission because seroconversion may take 6 to 8 weeks and the virus can be transmitted in residual leukocytes, so leukodepletion may also be carried out. CMV negative blood is recommended for low-birth-weight neonates, transplant patients, pregnant women, fetuses, and patients who are immunocompromised. **Gamma radiation** is used for irradiated blood products (whole blood, packed RBCs, platelets, plasma, and granulocytes) in order to destroy T-lymphocytes, which can proliferate in the recipient and attack the patient's organs as part of transfusion-associated graft vs host disease. Patients at risk include those who are immunocompromised, older adults, fetuses, neonates, patients receiving radiation or chemotherapy treatments, and those with leukemias, lymphomas, or other hematological cancers.

ABO DISCREPANCIES

ABO discrepancies occur when forward testing (RBC) does not match reverse testing (serum). Discrepancies can affect either forward and/or reverse testing. Reactions may be too weak or absent, or unexpected reactions may occur. ABO discrepancies may occur because of technical mistakes in carrying out the procedures or because of actual abnormalities of RBCs or serum. Discrepancies between forward and reverse groupings include:

- Group I: Reaction is weak or antibodies are absent.
- Group II: Antigens are absent instead of antibodies.
- Group III: Abnormalities are present in protein or plasma (increased globulin levels) associated with some diseases, such as Hodgkin lymphoma, or from Rouleaux formation (RBC aggregation with RBCs stacked in chains, which occurs with high levels of acute phase proteins (such as fibrinogen), paraproteinemias (amyloidosis, multiple myeloma) and some IV solutions (Dextran and PVP).
- Group IV: A variety of problems may occur because of autoantibodies, alloantibodies, and previous transfusions and bone marrow transplantation, including mixed field agglutination in which 2 different populations of cells are noted.

ABO discrepancies often occur during crossmatching:

- <u>Rouleaux formation</u>: Should disperse with serum dilution with normal saline. If still evident, aggregation represents hemagglutination. Note: Dilution may result in inability to detect weak antibodies.
- <u>Autoagglutination</u>: Reaction occurs in auto-control tube and may indicate the presence of cold agglutinins, autoantibodies, and alloantibodies. <u>Cold agglutinins</u> (anti-I, H, M, N, P, and Lewis) cause hemoagglutination at room temperature, but the reaction ceases at 37°C (confirming cold agglutinins). Complete antibody screen, and warm plasma and reagent RBCs for 15 minutes at 37°C and then carry out reverse ABO testing to eliminate interference of autoantibodies and <u>alloantibodies</u> (of foreign RBCs). <u>Autoantibodies,</u> most often produced in response to hemolytic anemias, frequently result in a positive direct antihuman globulin (AHG) test because of the autoantibodies coating the RBCs. The presence of autoantibodies is confirmed by washing the cells with NS, eluting the RBCs, and testing antisera. No agglutination should be noted.

TYPES OF IMMUNE RESPONSE

There are 2 different types of **immune response**:

- <u>Innate</u> (first line of defense): Available at birth as a first-line nonspecific defense against foreign pathogens and able to respond rapidly because it is not antigen dependent. The innate immune response includes barriers, such as the skin (epithelial cells), body oils (acidic), mucus (acidic), and stomach acid. In addition to barriers, the innate response includes an inflammatory response with phagocytosis (macrophages, neutrophils, dendritic cells). Natural killer cells kill pathogens. Mast cells stimulate cytokine production. The innate immune response activates the adaptive response.
- <u>Activated</u> (second line of defense): Involves the antigen-antibody responses. B-lymphocytes stimulate the humoral response (antibody production) and T-lymphocytes the cell-mediated response (antigens attacked and lymphokines secreted. Initially develops slowly as antibodies form in response to foreign antigen, but antibodies stay in the system and can be mobilized quickly with subsequent exposure.

ANTIBODY PRODUCTION

Antibody production: B cells contain antigen receptors (BCRs) and T-cells contain antigen receptor (TCR). Immunoglobulins (globular glycoproteins) are antibodies that can bind to antigens as part of activated immune response. Immunoglobulins are found in body fluids and on the surface of B cells. When the B cells are activated by contact with an antigen, the B cells proliferate and begin to differentiate into plasma cells, which produce antibodies:

- IgG—75-80%: Can be transported across the placenta and is the main immunoglobulin produced for secondary immune response and the only one with anti-toxin activity. Present in mucous membranes.
- IgA—15-20%: Primary antibody at mucous membranes where it prevents antigens from entering the immune system rather than destroying them.
- IgM—5-10%. Primarily found in peripheral circulation and is the main immunoglobulin produced for primary response and may be the only antibody produced against some antigens. Present on most mature B cells.
- IgD—0.2%: Found with IgM on many B cells, and its function is not yet clear.
- IgE—Trace. Most is bound to mast cells and basophils and is associated with allergic response.

IMMUNE DESTRUCTION OF RED CELLS BY HEMOLYSIS

Hemolysis occurs when the cell membrane is breached and hemoglobin is released into plasma. Intravascular hemolysis, which occurs within blood vessels, may result from inherited diseases (G6PD), acquired disease (DIC, TTP), autoimmune disorders, cardiac valvular prostheses, toxins (drugs, snakebite), parasitic disorders, and incompatible transfusions. RBC fragments or schistocytes are observed on peripheral smear. Extravascular hemolysis (most common), which happens outside of the blood vessels, occurs when antibodies attach to RBCs or the RBCs have abnormal morphology and are attacked prematurely and destroyed by phagocytosis in the spleen and liver. Mildly abnormal RBCs may be destroyed in the spleen (which can also sequester RBCs), but the liver has a superior blood supply and is able to more effectively destroy markedly abnormal RBCs. Hemolysis may result from a number of different pathogens, especially gram-positive microorganisms such as staphylococci, streptococci, and enterococci. Microspherocytes are observed on peripheral smear.

ACUTE PHASE REACTION

The **acute phase reaction** is part of the innate immune response when disturbance, such as infection or trauma, occurs. Phases include:

- Injury causes mononuclear phagocyte activation.
- Pro-inflammatory cytokines (glucocorticoids and nitric acid) released.
- Inflammatory cells activated.
- Hypothalamic-pituitary axis activated, resulting in changes in blood chemistry and fever, loss of appetite, and changes in sleep patterns.
- Vascular permeability and adhesiveness increase. Both prostaglandin synthesis and procoagulant activity increase.
- Liver increases production of acute phase proteins: C-reactive protein (CRP), serum amyloid A, haptoglobin, natural opsonin (MBL), complement proteins (C-3, C-4), ceruloplasmin, ferritin, fibrinogen. These proteins bind to microorganisms, modulate the immune response, binds to erythrocytes, and increases clot formation.

- Liver decreases production of storage and transport proteins (transferrin, albumin, transthyretin). The decrease in albumin and transferrin reduces the amount of iron available for microbial growth.
- Muscle and bone tissue breaks down.
- ESR increases because of increased plasma proteins (fibrinogen, immunoglobulins).

PRESENCE OF MUCINOUS GLYCOPROTEIN TUMOR MARKERS EXAMPLES

Cases in which the following mucinous glycoprotein tumor markers can be found in the human body:

1. CA 125: elevated in cases of lung cancer, pancreatic cancer, colon cancer, ovarian cancer, endometrial cancer, and metastatic breast cancer
2. CA 19-9: elevated in cases of colon cancer, chronic and acute pancreatitis, gastric cancer, hepatobiliary cancer, and pancreatic cancer
3. CA 15-3: elevated in pregnant and lactating women and in cases of breast cancer, lung cancer, liver cancer, stomach cancer, pancreatic cancer, and ovarian cancer; diminished in cases of tuberculosis, chronic hepatitis, lupus, cirrhosis, and sarcoidosis

COMPLEMENT SYSTEM

1. Opsonization: the improvement of a particle's phagocytosis after the attachment of C3b and IgG
2. Chemotaxis: process in which the presence of the anaphylatoxin C5a spurs the migration of monocytes and neutrophils
3. Immune adherence: process in which C3b attaches to immune complexes and other bodies
4. Kinin activation: process in which C2b reacts with C1, resulting in pain, smooth muscle contractions, elevated vascular permeability, and mucous gland secretion
5. Anaphylatoxins: the members of the complement system C3a, C4a, C5a; these substances encourage the release of histamine by mast cells and basophils; in addition, they increase vascular permeability and enable smooth muscle contractions

COMPLEMENT(S) DEFICIENT IN RECURRENT BACTERIAL INFECTION, COLLAGEN DISEASE, NEISSERIA INFECTION, ANGIOEDEMA, AND MASSIVE INFECTION

1. Recurrent bacterial infection: complements H or I will decrease
2. Collagen disease: complements C4, C2, or C1 will decrease
3. Neisseria infection: complements C5, C6, or C7 will decrease
4. Angioedema: complement C11NH will decrease
5. Massive infection: complement C3 will decrease

AUTOIMMUNE DISEASE

Any condition in which a person creates antibodies for their own antigens is an autoimmune disease. There are a couple of different theories that seek to explain autoimmune disease. The immunologic deficiency theory asserts that all of the antibodies produced by B lymphocytes are suppressed by T lymphocytes, and so antibodies are produced any time there is a decrease in T lymphocyte activity. The forbidden-clone theory asserts that occasionally lymphocytes erroneously fail to destroy autoantigens during fetal development. The theory of sequestered antigens asserts that some antigens can remain invisible to the immune system until tissue is damaged.

TYPE I HYPERSENSITIVITY

An immediate hypersensitivity is referred to as a type I hypersensitivity. This is simply an allergic reaction that occurs within minutes of contact with the allergen or antigen. An individual

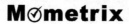

experiencing such a reaction is producing an increased level of IgE immunoglobulin. There are a few different laboratory tests that can be used to determine allergies by measuring total serum IgE: ELISA, RIST, RIA, and RAST.

Blood Banking and Transfusion Services

BLOOD BANKING TERMINOLOGY

Packed red blood cells	Red blood cell concentrate with most of the plasma removed. A 350 mL unit usually contains about 200 mL of RBCs and 30 mL of plasma along with 100 mL of a crystalloid solution. A few white blood cells and platelets may remain.
Irradiated red blood cells and platelets	Gamma irradiation of blood products inactivates T lymphocytes, which may cause graft vs host disease. Some RBCs are destroyed but platelet function is retained.
Washed red blood cells	Washing of RBC with 0.9% saline is done in a blood processor or centrifuge to remove plasma, plasma proteins, antibiotics, and other components in order to reduce risk of allergic reaction. However, this procedure results in 10-20% loss of RBCs and shelf-life is reduced to 4 hours if stored at 20°-24°C or 24 hours at 1°-6°C.
Frozen (glycerolized red blood cells	Glycerol is added to red blood cells through a filter. The glycerolized red blood cells are then spun in a centrifuge and concentrated. The RBCs can then be frozen for up to 10 years.
Deglycerolized red blood cells	Frozen plasma is thawed and "washed" to remove glycerol, which is added when RBCs are frozen but can result in hemolysis if it remains in the RBCs during transfusion.
Leukocyte reduction	T lymphocytes are removed from packed RBCs by centrifugation or filtration to reduce incidence of graft vs host disease in recipient.
Whole blood units	Contains all the blood components. One unit is approximately 450 to 500 mL.
HLA antigens	Human leukocyte antigens are major histocompatibility proteins on the surface of WBCs and are used for tissue typing.
Cryoprecipitate (antihemophilic factor)	Pooled units of plasma containing fibrinogen and other antihemophilic factors used to treat bleeding disorders, such as hemophilia.
Fresh frozen plasma	Plasma is frozen within 6 hours of donation and thawed for administration to control bleeding or to replace plasma. One unit (250 mL) of FFP is derived from 1 unit of whole blood and maintains clotting factors but is free of RBCs, WBCs, and platelets.
Platelet transfusion	Centrifugation separates platelet rich plasma (PRP) from whole blood and the PRP is further centrifugated to remove all but 50-60 mL plasma. Platelet transfusions may be from 1 donor (apheresis) or pooled donors (usually 6). Used for thrombocytopenia, CNS trauma, and patients on ECMO or cardiopulmonary bypass.
Anticoagulants	Products, such as EDTA and heparin, which prevent blood from clotting.

Product pooling	Products, such as plasma, pooled together from multiple screened donors, and cleansed to dissolve viruses.

PLASMAPHERESIS, PLATELETPHERESIS, AND LEUKAPHERESIS.

1. Plasmapheresis: form of hemapheresis in which plasma alone is removed from the blood of the donor; remaining blood products are returned to the donor, who may undergo this process once every eight weeks
2. Plateletpheresis: only platelets are removed from donor blood; performed with an electronic apheresis instrument; donors may undergo this process once every 48 hours
3. Leukapheresis: white blood cells alone are removed from donor blood; performed with electronic apheresis instrument; donors may undergo this process no more than twice a week or 24 times in one year

MAJOR CROSSMATCH, COMPATIBLE CROSSMATCH, AND INCOMPATIBLE CROSSMATCH

1. Major cross match: required test before a transfusion; donor cells tested with serum of potential recipient; antibodies come from serum, antigens come from donor cells
2. Compatible cross match: mixture of recipient's blood and donor cells produces no hemolysis or agglutination of cells
3. Incompatible cross match: mixture of blood of recipient and donor cells produces hemolysis and agglutination

GENERAL MOLECULAR STRUCTURE OF AN ANTIBODY

Every antibody has four molecular chains, two light chains and two heavy chains. The light chains contain a variable region in which the antibody bonding site is found. Some antibodies produce agglutination because of their reactions with the antigens on red blood cells. The heavy chains, on the other hand, determine the antibody's immunoglobulin type

ANTIBODY ENHANCER

An antibody enhancer is the chemical that stimulates the formation of antigen-antibody complexes. For instance, the proteolytic enzymes papain, ficin, and bromelain are frequently used as antibody enhancers, because they increase red blood cell agglutination. Bovine albumin, on the other hand, encourages sensitized red blood cells to form agglutination lattices. Low ionic strength solution, known by the abbreviation LISS, is often used to stimulate the formation of antigen-antibody complexes. Finally, polyethylene glycol additive, or PEG, concentrates antibodies.

HUMAN LEUKOCYTE ANTIGENS

Human leukocyte antigens (HLA) exist on both tissue cells and white blood cells, and are encoded by genes in the Major Histocompatibility Complex (MHC). This complex is found on the number six chromosome. For transfusions to be successful, human leukocyte antigens must be the same between donor and recipient for all stem cell, tissue, organ, and bone marrow donations. Otherwise, graft versus host disease is likely. Chills and fevers are the most common immune response to the presence of human leukocyte antigens.

ANTIGEN-ANTIBODY INTERACTIONS AND WAYS ANTIGEN-ANTIBODY COMPLEXES ARE HELD TOGETHER

The interactions between antigens and antibodies may result in the formation of a complex. An antigen will bond to the variable region on the light molecular chain of a corresponding antibody. These interactions may be stronger or weaker depending on the compatibility of the antigens and the antibody. In vitro, the reactions between an antigen and an antibody cause agglutination or hemolysis; in vivo, they may result in an immune response. The following forces conspire to hold together antigen-antibody complexes: hydrophobic bonding, hydrogen bonding, electrostatic charge, and Van der Waal's force.

GRADES OF AGGLUTINATION REACTIONS

Red blood cells can manifest six grades of agglutination reaction:

1. zero: lowest grade; no agglutinative red blood cells are present
2. $+^w$: red blood cell button divides into almost invisible or invisible clumps
3. 1+: red blood cell button divides into a number of small and medium-sized clumps
4. 2+: red blood cell button divides into numerous medium-sized clumps
5. 3+: red blood cell button divides into large clumps
6. 4+: red blood cell button does not break into clumps; free red blood cells cannot be seen in the background

ABO BLOOD SYSTEM

The ABO blood system differentiates based on the amount of A antigens and B antigens on the outside of red blood cells. Individuals who have red blood cells with both A and B antigens on the surface are said to have AB blood. This indicates that such individuals do not have antibodies (IgM) against these antigens in their blood serum. In like fashion, individuals who only have the B antigens on the surface are said to have B blood. Individuals will only have IgM antibodies against the A antigen. Similarly, individuals with type O blood will have red blood cells with neither A nor B antigens on the surface, but blood serum will contain antibodies against both A and B antigens.

FREQUENCIES OF O, A, B, AND AB BLOOD TYPES IN ETHNIC GROUPS

1. Asians: 40% type O; 28% type A; 27% type B; 5% type AB
2. Blacks: 49% type O; 27% type A; 20% type B; 4% type AB
3. Caucasians: 45% type O; 40% type A; 11% type B; 4% type AB

DETERMINING IF BLOOD TRANSFUSIONS WOULD BE SUCCESSFUL EXAMPLES

1. Donor type A, recipient type AB: successful transfusion, no agglutination
2. Donor type AB, recipient type A: unsuccessful transfusion, agglutination
3. Donor type O, recipient type B: successful transfusion, no agglutination; type O are universal donors
4. Donor type A, recipient type O: unsuccessful transfusion, agglutination
5. Donor type O, recipient type AB: successful transfusion, no agglutination; type AB are universal recipients

DETERMINING IF RECIPIENT/DONOR RELATIONSHIPS WOULD BE COMPATIBLE IN A MAJOR CROSS MATCH TEST EXAMPLES

1. Donor is O+ ; Recipient is A-: incompatible: recipients blood may contain anti-D antibodies, donors blood contains D antigens
2. Donor is A+ ; Recipient is AB+: compatible: recipients blood contains neither anti-A nor anti-B antibodies in serum, so donors blood is acceptable
3. Donor is A- ; Recipient is O-: incompatible: recipients blood contains both anti-A and anti-B antibodies in serum, so A antigens in the blood of donor will agglutinate
4. Donor is AB- ; Recipient is B-: incompatible: recipients blood contains anti-A antibodies in serum, which will agglutinate when mixed with A antigens

122

DETERMINING POSSIBLE BLOOD GENOTYPES AND PROBABILITY OF BLOOD TYPES FOR THE OFFSPRING EXAMPLES

1. Mother AB, father AO: offspring may have blood genotypes of AA, AB, AO, or BO; chance of type A is 50%, chance of type AB 25%, chance of type B 25%
2. Mother BO, father BO: possible genotypes BB, BO, or OO; chance of type B 75%, chance of type O 25%
3. Mother OO, father AO: possible genotypes AO, or OO; chance of type A 50%, chance of type O 50%
4. Mother AO, father BO: possible genotypes AB, BO, AO, OO; chance of type AB 25%, chance of type A 25% chance of type B 25%, chance of type O 25%

H ANTIGEN AS RELATED TO THE A, B, AND O BLOOD TYPES

The H antigen is part of the A and B antigens, functioning as an acceptor molecule for sugars. Blood type A is the H antigen with N-acetylgalactosamine affixed. Blood type B is H antigen with D-galactose affixed. Blood type B is also H antigen with no sugar affixed. Only .01% of the world's population has the h antigen rather than the H antigen, known as the Bombay blood group (phenotype hh). These individuals are universal donors because they lack A, B, and H antigens, but can only be transfused with Bombay blood group blood.

BLOOD GROUP SYSTEMS ABBREVIATIONS AND ANTIBODY CLASS

1. Kell: abbreviation K; antibody class IgG
2. Kidd: Jk; IgG
3. Duffy: Fy; IgG
4. Lutheran: Lu; IgG and IgM
5. Lewis: Le; IgM
6. P: P; IgM
7. MNS: MNS; IgG and IgM
8. Ii: I; IgM

BLOOD GROUP SYSTEMS ANTIGENS

1. Kell: K (kell), k (Cellano), Kpa, Kpb, Kpc, Jsa, Jsb, K11 (Cote), Wka, and Ku; the most common antigens are K12, K13, K16, K18, K19, K20, and K22
2. Duffy: Fya, Fyb, Fy3, Fy4, Fy5, and Fy6
3. Kidd: Jka, Jkb, and Jk3
4. MNS: M, N, S, s, and U; both of the M and N antigens are associated with glycophorin A; the S, s, and U antigens are associated with glycophorin B

BLOOD GROUP SYSTEM(S) OF RESISTANCE TO MALARIAL INFECTION, HEMOLYTIC DISEASE OF THE NEWBORN, *MYCOPLASMA PNEUMONIAE* INFECTION, CHRONIC GRANULOMATOUS DISEASE, PAROXYSMAL COLD HEMOGLOBINURIA

1. Resistance to malaria: Duffy blood group; phenotype Fy-a-b- is most resistant
2. Hemolytic disease of the newborn: related to Rh, ABO, Kell, MNS, and Duffy blood group systems
3. Infection with Mycoplasma pneumoniae: related to Ii blood group system
4. Chronic granulomatous disease: related to Kell blood group system, especially phenotype K-k-Kp(a-b-)
5. Paroxysmal cold hemoglobinuria: related to P blood group system, especially the Donath-Landsteiner antibody

DETERMINING IF THE MOTHER SHOULD RECEIVE A DOSAGE OF RHIG EXAMPLES

1. Rh positive mother, Rh negative baby: The mother is not a candidate for RhIg because she is Rh positive.
2. Rh negative mother, Rh negative baby: The mother is not a candidate for RhIg because even though she is Rh negative, she gave birth to a Rh negative baby.
3. Rh negative mother, D^u negative mother, Rh positive baby: The mother is a candidate for RhIg because she is Rh negative (D^u negative), and she gave birth to a Rh positive baby.
4. Rh negative mother, D^u negative mother, triplets (one is Rh positive, and two are Rh negative): The mother is a candidate for RhIg because she is Rh negative, and at least one of her triplets is a Rh positive baby.

PURPOSE OF A CROSSMATCH

Crossmatch tests are used to decrease the risk of negative transfusion reaction. However, cross matching is unable to locate viruses, bacteria, or parasites in the blood of the donor. Individuals may also suffer delayed transfusion reactions or allergic reactions, neither of which can be predicted with cross matching. Also, cross matching has no effect on the formation of antibodies to any foreign antigens in the red blood cells of the donor. For these reasons, cross matching is not a foolproof way to make transfusion safe.

REGULATION PARAMETERS FOR COMPUTER CROSSMATCH

Under 21 CFR 6096.15 (c), the FDA has established regulations for recipient-donor **computer crossmatch** for transfusions:

- User must be able to verify and accept or reject data.
- Data elements must include the recipient's unique ID number, RBC antibody screening, ABO/Rh (D) typing, sample, and special transfusion requirements (such as leukoreduction) and the donor's unique identification number, component name, ABO/Rh (D) blood type, special requirements and RBC antibody screening.
- Written procedures should outline decision tables and decision rules.
- The system should provide warning messages when actions are out of conformance with decision rules.
- User validation tests must be run on all new equipment/processes in the same environment in which they will be utilized and re-validation carried out according to written program.
- Records must be maintained for all compatibility tests, calibration, equipment standardization, and performance checks for at least 10 years.
- Implementation of computer crossmatch or change in procedure as allowed under licensure must be reported to the FDA.
- Unvalidated systems must undergo testing to meet requirements for validation.

PROSPECTIVE BLOOD DONOR EXAMINATION

The following are the basic examinations and requirements for prospective blood donors:

- temperature: lower than 99.5°F
- blood pressure: lower than 180/100
- pulse: between 50 and a hundred beats per minute
- body weight: at least 110 pounds
- hematocrit: at least 38%
- hemoglobin: at least 12.5 g/dL

Example exclusion periods:

1. Malaria: three years following last infection
2. Taking aspirin: none for whole blood; 48-72 hours for platelet donation
3. Viral hepatitis: permanent deferral
4. Accutane use: one month after last use
5. Exposure to the blood of another person: one month following exposure
6. Taken clotting factors in the past: permanent deferral
7. Male prospective donor who has had sex with another male: one year from last sexual contact with a male

DETERMINING IF DONATING WHOLE BLOOD IS POSSIBLE EXAMPLES

1. A 33-year-old woman with a hematocrit of 38: allowed to donate whole blood at present; hematocrit is above minimum acceptable level of 36
2. A 48-year-old man who received a blood transfusion 5 months ago: not able to donate whole blood at present; recent blood transfusion creates possibility of hepatitis transmission; hepatitis B has an incubation period of six months
3. A 21-year-old woman who received a tattoo 14 months ago: able to donate whole blood at present; individuals are not allowed to donate blood within 12 months of receiving a tattoo
4. A 35-year-old man who went on a trip to Nigeria 3 months ago: not allowed to donate blood at present; individuals who do not take a prophylactic for malaria before visiting Africa may donate within six months of their return; individuals who do take a prophylactic must wait three years from their return

AUTOLOGOUS DONATION

An autologous donation of blood is one in which an individual donates blood for their own personal use in future transfusions. This system eliminates the possibility of a negative transfusion reaction or the passage of disease. On the other hand, autologous donations are expensive and can be wasteful of blood. There are four kinds of autologous donation: preoperative donation, intraoperative collection, intraoperative hemodilution, and postoperative collection.

PROCEDURE FOR DRAWING BLOOD

The procedure for **drawing blood from donors** includes:

1. Verifying identification.
2. Using standard precautions and standard venipuncture protocols.
3. Drawing blood from an antecubital vein if possible using a sterile collection unit comprised of a large gauge (16-18) needle connected to a closed system with drainage tube and collection bag.
4. Allowing the collection bag to fill with blood by gravity by placing the bag in a mixing unit below the level of the arm. The collection bag contains an anticoagulant to prevent clotting and a preservative, such as CPD. The citrate prevents clots from forming, the phosphate stabilizes the blood pH, and the dextrose provides nutrients to the cells.
5. Checking the weight of collection bag to determine when it is filled (usually at about 450 mL).
6. Securing the collection bag and removing the needle.
7. Note: If for some reason the blood flow stops, a complete new setup and collection unit must be used if further blood is taken from the donor as only 1 needle puncture can be used per unit.

POSSIBLE DONOR ADVERSE REACTIONS

On occasion, an individual will experience an adverse reaction when donating blood. Fainting, nausea, rapid breathing, and dizziness are all common side effects of donation. When these or more severe side effects, like convulsions or heart trouble, occur, the tech should immediately remove the tourniquet and blood collection bag. Cold compresses and smelling salts may be appropriate. In especially severe cases, one should make sure that the individual's airway is open and that his or her pulse rate is normal.

CONFIDENTIAL UNIT EXCLUSION

In the process known as confidential unit exclusion, blood donors are allowed to select whether they want their blood products to be discarded or used again for future transfusions. The donor is asked to select a label with a bar code indicating whether or not the blood products should be used in the future; it is impossible to tell by any other means than scanning the barcode what decision the donor has made.

LABEL REQUIREMENTS FOR ALL DONATED BLOOD PRODUCTS

Donated blood products must have a label with the following information: contents; amount of blood collected; volume of blood collected; expiration date; unique number for that particular donated unit; ABO and D type of the blood component; donor classification; prescription requirements; warning regarding infectious agents; FDA license number; information regarding the Circular of Information; type and amount of anticoagulant; and recommended storage temperature.

PREPARING RED BLOOD CELLS, PLATELETS, AND PLASMA FROM WHOLE BLOOD

Using a centrifuge, lab technicians can separate whole blood into red blood cells, platelets, and plasma. The process is as follows: the bag of whole blood is placed in the centrifuge, immediately separating red blood cells from plasma and platelets. These red blood cells are placed into a separate bag, at which point an additive solution may be mixed in. Plasma and platelets are put into a platelet pack, which is then centrifuged again, separating platelets from plasma. Plasma is put into a fresh frozen plasma bag, while platelets remain in the original container.

ELUTION AND TYPES OF ELUTION TECHNIQUES

One process that can remove antibodies that are fixed to red blood cells in vivo is called elution. There are three basic kinds of elution:

- Lui freeze-thaw technique: IgM antibodies are removed from the red blood cells of newborn babies
- Digitonin destroys the red blood cells, releasing antibodies
- Intact red blood cell antibody removal (RES): red blood cells are not destroyed, but antibodies are removed using buffers

PREWARMED TECHNIQUE FOR AVOIDING COLD ANTIBODIES

One of the ways that lab technicians try to avoid cold antibodies is by using what is known as the prewarmed technique. This technique is performed as follows: a drop of panel cells and auto control cells is put into a test tube, which is then warmed for 10 minutes at 37°C. Simultaneously, a tube of serum from the patient is warmed for 10 minutes at 37°C. The serum is then added to the warmed panel cells, and the mixture continues to incubate for 30 minutes. At this point, it is washed three times with saline that has been heated to 37°C. Finally, antihuman globulin is added and the reactions of the materials can be interpreted.

EXAMPLE SITUATIONS WHERE TRANSFUSIONS WOULD BE INDICATED

1. Red blood cells: before surgery, radiation therapy, or chemotherapy; after trauma; for sickle cell anemia; for premature infants
2. Platelets: during excessive post operation bleeding; during chemotherapy; after a bone marrow transplant
3. Plasma: liver disease coupled with bleeding; abnormal coagulation reaction after transfusion; before surgery for those already taking anticoagulant drugs
4. Whole blood: individuals who've lost 25% or more of the entire blood volume; exchange transfusion

EXAMPLE SITUATIONS WHERE BLOOD PRODUCTS WOULD BE USED

1. Washed red blood cells: infant and intrauterine transfusions; for individuals who suffer anaphylactic, allergic, or febrile reactions to donated plasma proteins
2. Leukocyte-reduced red blood cells: chronically transfused patients
3. Irradiated red blood cells: bone marrow transplants, progenitor cell transplants, during chemotherapy or radiation therapy, and during intrauterine transfusions; occasionally given to immunodeficient individuals or premature infants

MINIMAL REQUIREMENTS (TRANSFUSION TRIGGERS) FOR TRANSFUSION OF RED BLOOD CELLS

RBC Hgb transfusion trigger	Transfusions
<6 g/dL	In almost all circumstances
6-7 g/dL	In most circumstances
Septic shock >6 hours @7 g/dL	Generally indicated
Septic shock <6 hours @ 8 g/dL	Generally indicated
Cardiac or orthopedic surgery, 7-8 g/dL	May be indicated, depending on condition.
Oncologic or hematologic-associated thrombocytopenia, acute coronary artery syndrome, continuing bleeding @8-10 g/dL	May be indicated, depending on condition and risks.
>10 g/dL	Usually not indicated

CRYOPRECIPITATE TRANSFUSION TRIGGERS

- Adults: Surgical bleeding, severe hemorrhage, post-cardiac surgery hemorrhage.
- Neonates: Factor VIII, XIII deficiencies, von Willebrand disease, congenital fibrinogen deficiency.

FRESH FROZEN PLASMA TRANSFUSION TRIGGERS

Fresh frozen plasma triggers depend on underlying condition:

- Acute DIC.
- Bleeding while receiving massive transfusion.
- Reversal of warfarin with intracranial hemorrhage.
- Fluid for apheresis replacement for TTP and HUS.
- Preprocedure prophylactic for those on warfarin if surgery is emergent.

PLATELETS TRANSFUSION TRIGGERS

Platelet transfusion triggers depend on underlying condition:

- Neonate: <20,000
- Neonate with active bleeding or undergoing invasive procedure: 20,000 to <30,000.
- Neonate with low birth weight, cerebral hemorrhage, sepsis, thrombocytopenia, coagulation disorders: 30,000 to 50,000.
- Adult, not actively bleeding but to undergo major surgery: ≤50,000.
- Adult, not actively bleeding but to undergo neurological or ocular surgery: ≤100,000.
- Adult, active bleeding and to undergo surgery: <50,000.
- Adult, not actively bleeding and stable: <10,000.
- Adult, not actively bleeding and stable but temperature elevated (>38°C) or to undergo invasive procedure: <20,000.

TRANSFUSION-TRANSMITTED INFECTIONS

Viruses	Bacteria/Prion	Parasites
Hepatitis A virus (rare)	Bacteria (Contamination):	Malaria (*Plasmodium* spp.)
Hepatitis B virus	*Staphylococcus aureus*	Chagas (*Trypanosoma cruzi*)
Hepatitis C virus	*Anaplasma*	Babesiosis (*Babesia microti*)
Hepatitis E virus (rare)	*phagocytophilum*	Leishmaniasis (*Leishmania*
Human immunodeficiency virus	*Rickettsia rickettsii.*	*donovani*)
(HIV)	*Yersinia enterocolitica*	
Human T-lymphotropic virus	*Escherichia coli*	
West Nile virus	*Klebsiella, Proteus,*	
Cytomegalovirus	*Acinetobacter*	
Human herpesvirus 8	Prion:	
Parvovirus B19	Variant Creutzfeldt-Jacob	
SARS-CoV virus	disease (CJD)	
H5N1 influenza virus		
Dengue virus (DENV)		
Zika virus (ZIKV)		
Chikungunya virus (CHIKV)		

LOOK-BACK/RECALL PROCEDURES FOR BLOOD PRODUCTS

Look-back procedures are triggered when a transfusion recipient becomes infected and all donors are traced or a donor is discovered to have an infection and all recipients are traced. For donors who convert to positive for HIV, recipients of any component within the previous 12 months must be notified by the hospital or physician. For donors who convert to positive for hepatitis C virus, the recipient or physician must be notified. The physician can make the decision about notifying the recipient. **Recall of blood products** occurs when additional information becomes available about the donor, but in many cases the products have already been transfused and the recipients must be located. The FDA issues recalls and specific directions for look-back, such as the look-back time period. Recall classifications include:

- Class I: Adverse health consequences or death likely.
- Class II: Temporary or reversible adverse health consequences may occur.
- Class III: Very little risk of adverse health consequences.

ROUTINE AND EMERGENT TRANSFUSION ADMINISTRATION PROTOCOL

Routine transfusion procedure:

- Obtain blood product after IV access is in place.
- Verify labels, and blood typing with another nurse or physician.
- Examine blood product for visual evidence of hemolysis or contamination.
- Initiate within correct time period and infuse for specified time and at specified rate.
- Monitor patient carefully over first 30 minutes, including vital signs as per protocol.
- Change tubing for PRBCs every 2 hours and flush tubing with NS after administration of FFP or platelets.

Emergent transfusion procedure:

- Administer type O, Rh+ red blood cells to adult males and adult females of non-child bearing age/potential.
- Change to type O, Rh+ red blood cells (except for females of child-bearing age) if >6 units needed in 24 hours and type specific blood is not available.
- Administer type O, Rh- red blood cells to pediatric patients and females of child-bearing age/potential.
- Provide type specific blood as soon as typing and crossmatching are completed.
- If blood supply is limited, maintain and use only type O, Rh-blood for emergent situations.

TRANSFUSION REACTION INVESTIGATION

Transfusion reaction investigations are carried out in response to acute transfusion reactions (mild to severe), delayed, and suspected reactions. The procedure for transfusion reaction investigation includes:

1. Obtain clotted and anticoagulated post-transfusion blood samples for the blood bank/center.
2. Take blood product, transfusion set, and IV solution to blood bank/center.
3. Review labels, IV fluid (saline), pre-and post-transfusion samples, records, and test results.
4. Visually check blood product for signs of contamination and/or hemolysis (note color change) and compare with pre-transfusion samples.
5. Note evidence of post-transfusion plasma hemoglobin and hemoglobinuria.
6. Culture blood product.
7. Conduct patient laboratory investigation: leukocyte count, BNP, HLA class I and II antigens.
8. Obtain first urine sample after reaction and then a 24-hour sample.
9. Repeat blood typing (ABO Rh[D]) to ensure the product was labeled correctly and administered to the correct patient.
10. Compare results of post-transfusion blood typing with pre-transfusion typing and repeat of the procedure if disparities are evident.

Based on the results of the investigation, if an error occurred, the staff must be educated about the error and procedures instituted to avoid further errors.

STEPS TO TAKE BEFORE STARTING A TRANSFUSION AND IF A TRANSFUSION REACTION IS SUSPECTED

Before a transfusion is begun, the lab technician should double-check the tag on the blood bag as well as the paperwork associated with the requisition. During a blood transfusion, the individual's vital signs should be checked every quarter hour. Vital signs that must be checked include body temperature, pulse, blood pressure, and respiration. If a transfusion reaction begins or is suspected, the transfusion should stop immediately. The patient's physician should then be notified.

ANAPHYLACTIC TRANSFUSION REACTIONS

An anaphylactic transfusion reaction begins almost immediately after a transfusion is initiated. This is a kind of allergic reaction that manifests with bronchospasms, wheezing, and cough, but no fever. Anaphylactic transfusion reaction can be fatal if not treated immediately. It is caused by a genetic deficiency in IgA antibodies.

DELAYED HEMOLYTIC TRANSFUSION REACTIONS

A delayed hemolytic transfusion reaction typically occurs five to seven days after the transfusion. Symptoms may include fever or mild jaundice. This kind of transfusion reaction is slightly more common than acute hemolytic transfusion reaction, but does not usually pose a threat to survival. The following laboratory tests indicate a possible delayed hemolytic transfusion reaction: positive antibody screen post-transfusion; positive direct antiglobulin test; decreased level of hematocrit; and decreased level of hemoglobin.

ACUTE HEMOLYTIC TRANSFUSION REACTIONS

An acute hemolytic transfusion reaction happens immediately after the transfusion. Possible symptoms include fever, tachycardia, hemoglobinemia, hypotension, and chills. This severe reaction may be the result of incompatible transfusions or reactions between antibodies and antigens. Although acute hemolytic transfusion reactions are quite rare, they are potentially deadly. The following are indications that such a reaction may be occurring: decreased haptoglobin, elevated bilirubin, and elevated plasma free hemoglobin.

SENSITIZATION IN RELATION TO ANTIGEN-ANTIBODY REACTIONS

In many in vitro antigen-antibody reactions, the first stage is sensitization, the point at which the antibody has attached to the antigen but has not yet produced any agglutination or hemolysis. The optimal pH for sensitization is 7. The degree of sensitization will depend on incubation time, defined as the amount of time in which the antibody has to attach to the antigens. Also, antibodies will react most strongly at a temperature of 37°C. Finally, sensitization will be increased in proportion to the ratio of serum to cells; more serum means more available antibodies.

IMMUNE-MEDIATED NONHEMOLYTIC TRANSFUSION REACTIONS

Immune-mediated nonhemolytic transfusion reactions occur when the recipient has HLA antibodies that react to the donor's antigens and cytokines. This condition manifests in back pain, headache, nausea, vomiting, and a fever beginning age to 24 hours after the transfusion. This condition is especially common in women who have undergone multiple pregnancies or other individuals who have undergone multiple transfusions. This condition occurs in approximately 1 out of every 200 donor units.

GRAFT VERSUS HOST DISEASE

Graft versus host disease is a rare condition that occurs when T cells from a donor react to the cells of the recipient. This condition typically emerges between 3 and 30 days after the transfusion and may manifest as abnormal liver function, erythromatous maculopapular rash, and fever. Sepsis and even death can result from untreated graft versus host disease.

HEMOLYTIC DISEASE OF THE NEWBORN

When the IgG antibodies of a pregnant mother travel through the placenta and attack the red blood cells of the fetus, the ensuing condition is called hemolytic disease of the newborn. There are two results: the fetus may become anemic, leading to heart failure; hemoglobin from destroyed red blood cells is converted into indirect bilirubin, leading to jaundice. This latter result can lead to intellectual disability, brain damage, deafness, and in some cases, death.

RH HEMOLYTIC DISEASE OF THE NEWBORN VS. ABO HEMOLYTIC DISEASE OF THE NEWBORN

The most severe form of hemolytic disease of the newborn is Rh hemolytic disease of the newborn. This form of the disease occurs when a D negative mother develops D antibodies in response to a D positive baby. If the same mother subsequently has another D positive baby, the D antibodies from the first pregnancy may attack the red blood cells of the second baby. It is often necessary to perform an exchange transfusion to mitigate symptoms of this disease. Another kind of hemolytic disease of the newborn is ABO hemolytic disease, which occurs in babies with blood type A or B who have mothers with blood type O. ABO hemolytic disease can be treated with phototherapy, to remove excess bilirubin.

PREVENTING HEMOLYTIC DISEASE OF THE NEWBORN

Hemolytic disease of the newborn can be prevented in the following ways:

- A pregnant D negative mother can be given 300 micrograms of prenatal Rh immune globulin at 28 weeks
- D negative women who have had abortions, amniocentesis, percutaneous umbilical blood sampling, abdominal trauma, intrauterine transfusion, or ectopic pregnancies should be given 300 micrograms of Rh immune globulin
- D negative women can be given 300 micrograms of Rh immune globulin within 72 hours after delivery

DIRECT ANTIGLOBULIN TEST (DAT)

The direct antiglobulin test (DAT) detects either IgG antibodies in their blood sample or complement proteins affixed to red blood cells. The test is performed as follows: red blood cells are washed three times with a saline solution, after which antihuman globulin is added. Agglutination at this point indicates the presence of either complement proteins or IgG antibodies. A DAT is often performed in cases of hemolytic disease of the newborn, autoimmune hemolytic anemia, or transfusion reaction.

INDIRECT ANTIGLOBULIN TEST

The indirect antiglobulin test (IAT) measures the sensitization of red blood cells in vitro. The test is performed as follows: patient's blood serum is mixed with red blood cells and incubated at body temperature. Once the IgG antibodies in the serum have had a chance to attach to the red blood cells, the mixture is washed and antihuman globulin is added. Any agglutination indicates IgG antibodies. A false negative may occur when the washing is not done properly or when antihuman globulin is not added to the solution. A false positive may occur when red blood cells are agglutinated before being washed.

DONATH-LANDSTEINER (D-L) TEST

The Donath-Landsteiner test indicates whether paroxysmal cold hemoglobinuria is present. When this condition is present, individuals will contain hemoglobin cold temperatures. The roots of this disorder are in the anti-P antibody of the P blood group system. This antibody connects to the surfaces of red blood cells in temperatures below 37°C and at warmer temperatures causes hemolysis. The Donath-Lansteiner test is performed as follows: a test tube of serum and red blood cells is placed at 4°C, while a control to his place at 37°C. The test tube of serum and blood is gradually warmed to 37°C, at which point the tubes are centrifuged. If after centrifuging neither displays an indication of hemolysis, the test is negative. When the tube containing serum and red blood cells shows evidence of hemolysis, but the control tube does not, the test is positive. If both tubes show evidence of hemolysis, the test is rendered invalid.

BLOOD LABELING REQUIREMENTS

The FDA requires that all blood products and materials used for transfusion be labeled with machine-readable **labeling language** to decrease incidence of errors related to the wrong patient or wrong product. The label must contain at least the unique facility ID, the donor's lot number, the product code, and the blood type of the donor. The two labeling languages in use include:

- Codabar: Labeling that includes an identifying barcode, a description of the contents (such as "RED BLOOD CELLS"), the volume, additives, storage requirements, and test results of FDA required tests (such as HIV and HBV.
- ISB-128: The international standard for identification and labeling as well as transfer of information about body products, including blood. ISB-128 provides a standard terminology, reference tables to apply the appropriate codes, data structures, delivery mechanisms, and standard layout for labels.

TRANSFUSION RECORD DOCUMENTATION AND TRANSFUSION ADMINISTRATION PROTOCOL

Transfusion record documentation must be maintained for at least 5 years and those required for tracing a blood product from donor to disposition maintained for at least 10 years following administration or 5 years after expiration date. Computerized records must be secure and software validated. Records must include all those associated with the donor, recipient, and blood product, including testing (all steps and results), storage, and disposition. The records must be easily accessible and allow for tracing of blood products. Donor records must be maintained and should include information about storage temperatures and visual blood inspections, and preparation of components. Recipient records should include blood type and information regarding antibodies history of transfusions, and adverse transfusion reactions. Records should also be maintained regarding therapeutic phlebotomy, policies and procedures, cytapheresis procedures, antibody identification, quality control, and shipping.

MAINTAINING PROPER RECORDS OF ALL QUALITY CONTROL AND BLOOD BANK PROCEDURES

Proper **record keeping and documentation** for quality control and blood bank procedures are maintained at 4 different levels:

- Blood bank polices: A statement of intent that should include the principles that will be utilized to guide decision-making and procedures and may outline the roles and responsibility of employees as well as financial basis for maintaining the program. An example: Employee practices that ensure blood safety.
- Blood bank processes: These should outline the way things happen, including the chain of command and basic methods of dealing with various functions of the blood bank, such as collecting, storing, and distributing blood products.
- Blood bank procedures: These are step-by-step explanations of how each blood bank procedure, such as collecting a blood sample or applying a label to a blood product, is carried out, including the equipment and supplies needed.

- - Supporting documentation/Forms: These should include all forms of documentation that are required and samples to show the correct manner of completing and filling out forms required forms.

PROPER STORAGE AND TRANSPORTATION OF BLOOD AND BLOOD PRODUCTS FOR TRANSFUSIONS

The FDA and AAB have established temperature standards for storage and transportation of blood and blood products:

Product	Storage	Transportation
Whole blood, red blood cells (including irradiated, deglycerolized, leukocyte reduced, washed, apheresis), and plasma (including any form after thawing and liquid).	1° to 6°C	1° to 10°C
Platelets (any form), apheresis granulocytes (including irradiated), anti-hemophilic factor (including cryoprecipitated, thawed cryoprecipitated, and plasma thawed cryoprecipitated).	20° to 24°C with continuous agitation	20° to 24°C
Antihemophilic factor (including plasma cryoprecipitated, pooled cryoprecipitated before freezing), plasma (including frozen within 24 hours of phlebotomy and cryoprecipitate reduced).	≤-18°C	Frozen
Fresh frozen plasma	≤-18°C or ≤-65°C	≤-18°C or ≤-65°C

VISIBLE INSPECTION OF UNITS OF BLOOD/COMPONENTS

Contamination	Cryoprecipitate	Plasma	Platelets	RBCs
Bacteria	Bubbles, clot, fibrin strains, >opaque	Bubbles, clot, fibrin strains, >opaque	Bubbles, clot, fibrin strains, >opaque, grey appearance	Dk. Purple -> black
Bile	Bright yellow -> brown	Bright yellow -> brown	Bright yellow -> brown	----
Color abnormality	Any abnormal color	Any abnormal color	Any abnormal color	Supernatant grey/brown
Hemolysis	Pink -> red	Pink -> red	----	Bright red
Lipids	White appearance, > opaque	White appearance, > opaque	White appearance, >opaque	Lighter red, >opaque
Particulates	Clots, aggregates of cellular material	t, fibrin strands, white materials	Clot, fibrin strands, white materials	Clots, white materials
RBC contamination	Lt pink -> red	Lt pink -> red	Lt. pink	----

BLOOD BANK REGULATIONS

OSHA and state regulations outline the requirements for **disposition of blood bags and patient samples**. Blood disposition must comply with OSHA's Bloodborne Pathogen's Standard (29 CFR 1910.1030), which covers blood (semi-liquid, liquid, dried) in containers, in other waste products, or on items, such as sharps. As a regulated waste, the blood must be placed in a container that is closable, leak-proof, labeled (proper color-coding), and closed before removal to avoid any spillage or loss of contents during transport to disposal site. **Temperatures:** Blood bank refrigerators are maintained between 2° and 4°C with audible and visible alarm if the temperature falls to 6°C. Freezers are maintained at -20°C, with alerts when the temperature falls to -19°C. Incubators usually provide for a range of temperatures (5° to 70°C) with much incubation done at 37°C. The alarm system for refrigerators, freezers, and incubators should be battery powered so it still functions if the electrical supply is cut.

REQUIREMENTS FOR BLOOD BANK OPERATION

Requirements for blood bank operation include:

1. Obtaining a blood bank license and renewing annually.
2. Being available for inspection upon request.
3. Participating in proficiency testing.
4. Obtaining qualified director and adequate numbers of other qualified personnel.
5. Supervising staff, identifying training needs, and implementing training.
6. Having appropriate equipment for all functions.
7. Using appropriate infection control practices and disposing contaminated materials appropriately.
8. Carrying out a documented review for collection/preparation of all blood components.
9. Maintaining a manual that outlines all policies and procedures.
10. Maintaining correct and legible records that includes significant steps in procedures, test outcomes, ABO/Rh typing result, and donor records, and carrying out reporting responsibilities.
11. Establishing criteria for blood collection, processing, storage, distribution, and testing.
12. Labeling in compliance with Code of Federal Regulations.
13. Storing blood/blood components appropriately and at correct temperature with temperature monitoring system in place.

QUALITY CONTROL FOR ALL REAGENTS

Reagent solutions are used for most diagnostic tests, and results are often dependent on using the correct reagent (stock, working, or standard) at the correct concentration. Quality control procedures include ensuring:

- Accurate weighing and measuring when preparing reagent solutions.
- Carefully following of directions and/or using reagent kits when preparing reagent solutions.
- Choosing the correct reagent.
- Following recommended procedures when disposing of reagents.
- Using proper PPE when working with reagents.
- Neutralizing spilled acids/corrosive chemicals with sodium carbonate or sodium bicarbonate and alkali with dry sand.
- Labeling strong acids and alkali (corrosive compounds) and storing near the floor.

- Properly storing all reagents (acid in glass, flammable reagents in metal or glass, sodium/potassium hydroxide in plastic, hygroscopic chemicals in desiccator or air-tight container, photosensitive chemicals in dark, glass stoppered bottle).
- Monitoring volumes/concentration of chemicals that are explosive when dehydrated.
- Diluting stock only as needed.
- Labeling reagent solutions with date and other information according to directions.
- Labeling all poisonous, flammable, and otherwise hazardous materials.

OPTIMUM STORAGE TEMPERATURES

1. Frozen red blood cells: -65°C or less; 10 years from collection date
2. Platelets: between 20 and 24°C; five days from collection date
3. Cryoprecipitate: -18°C or less; one year after collection date
4. Pooled platelets: between 20 and 24°C; four hours after pooling
5. Thawed red blood cells: between one and 6°C; 24 hours after thawing

OPTIMUM STORAGE TEMPERATURE AND EXPIRATION DATES FOR RED BLOOD CELLS NOT FROZEN OR PREVIOUSLY FROZEN

Any red blood cells that have not been frozen should be stored at temperatures between one and 6 degrees Celsius. If CPD (citrate-phosphate-dextrose) or CP2D (citrate-phosphate-2-dextrose) is the anticoagulant, the expiration date for the red blood cells is three weeks after collection. However, if the anticoagulant is CPDA-1 (citrate-phosphate-dextrose-adenine-one), red blood cells can last five weeks. If the anticoagulants AS-1, AS-2, or AS-3 were used, the red blood cells will last six weeks after collection.

PROBLEM OF THE BACTERIAL CONTAMINATION OF BLOOD PRODUCTS

Occasionally, blood products in storage will suffer a bacterial contamination. The most common type of bacterial contaminant is *Yersinia enterocolitica*. Bacteria of this kind will grow while the product is being stored. Individuals who receive blood products that have been contaminated are likely to manifest symptoms similar to those of an adverse transfusion reaction: fever and chills, e.g. Clots, discoloration, or hemolysis in the blood unit indicates possible contamination.

TRANSPORTATION GUIDELINES FOR BLOOD PRODUCTS

Platelets should be transported at room temperature, and they should not be jostled. Red blood cells must be transported at a temperature between one and 10°C; it is standard to place red blood cells in a Styrofoam box inside a cardboard box and on ice. Frozen blood components must be shipped on dry ice and wrapped well.

PURPOSE AND CRITERIA FOR THERAPEUTIC PHLEBOTOMY

Therapeutic phlebotomy, a blood draw to treat disease, is commonly done to reduce concentration or numbers of red blood cells, ferritin (iron), or porphyrins in the blood for patients with:

- Polycythemia: Increased hemoglobin and hematocrit because of increased red blood cell count that makes blood more viscous.
- Hematochromatosis: Abnormal accumulation of iron in the body, leading to organ damage.
- Porphyrias: Group of disorders in which porphyrins (which are necessary for hemoglobin to function properly) build up in the body.

Blood, usually in about 500 mL units, is withdrawn in a similar manner to blood donations, but most blood is discarded although the FDA allows blood obtained through therapeutic phlebotomy for hematochromatosis to be donated. Patients will have therapeutic phlebotomy on a schedule ordered by the physician, usually to achieve a target hemoglobin. Some patients require blood draws every few days and others once monthly or less frequently.

SPECIAL REQUIREMENTS OF BLOOD PRODUCTS

Cytomegalovirus (CMV) negative transfusions: Blood is screened for anti-CMV antibodies and labeled as seronegative although this does not completely eliminate the risk that CMV will be transmitted because the donor's blood may contain CMV from a recent infection without showing antibodies. CMV negative blood is provided for patients who are immunocompromised, such as HIV patients, post-splenectomy patients, and donors for or recipients of bone marrow or stem cell transplants. CMV negative blood is also given for seronegative antepartum patients, low birth weight infants of seronegative mothers, and intrauterine transfusions.

Massive transfusions: Transfusions of 10 (trauma definition) or 20 (traditional definition) units in 24 hours (ratio of plasma to RBCs of 1:1 or 1:2+) for treatment of hemorrhage. Massive transfusions are indicated for loss of 50% of blood volume over a 3-hour period.

Baby units: Red blood cells for infants are prescribed in mL rather than units with the usual volume 5 mL/kg/h (this may be higher with active bleeding) and for platelets 10-20 mL/kg for children up to 15 kg and 300 mL for those over 15 kg.

Microbiology

BACTERIOLOGY TERMINOLOGY

Mesophilic	Organisms that grow best at moderate temperatures (20°-45°C).
Autotrophic	Self-nourishing organisms that can produce organic constituents from inorganic salts and carbon dioxide.
Semipermeable	Cell membranes that allow the passage of some materials though the membrane but not others.
Ambient	That found in the surroundings, such as ambient light.
Thermophilic	Organisms that grow best at extreme temperatures (41°-122°C).
Heterotopic	Normal cells found in abnormal location or displacement from normal location.
Bacteriophage	Virus that infects and lyses (disintegrates) bacteria.
Pathogenic	Disease-causing organism, such as virus, fungus, and bacterium.
Phagocytosis	Process in which phagocytes engulf other microorganisms, cells, or foreign particles to destroy them.
Bacteria	Single-cell prokaryotic microorganisms that come in a variety of shapes, including coccus (spheres), bacillus (rods), spirals (DNA-like), and filamentous (elongated).
Capsule	The outside polysaccharide layer that surrounds some types of bacteria and protects the cell and provides a virulence factor.
Cytoplasm	Gel-like substance in the interior of the cell that comprises water, enzymes, various nutrients, waste products, and cell structures.
Nucleoid	Strands of DNA found in the cytoplasm.
Cell wall / membrane	The cell wall is a subcapsular layer composed of peptidoglycan and is rigid to protect the underlying cytoplasmic membrane, which is composed of proteins and phospholipids that regulate the flow of substances to and from the cell. Composition varies among different bacteria. Gram-negative organisms have a thicker outer covering and gram-positive organisms have a thinner outer layer.
Spore	Resistant resting and/or reproductive stage of bacteria.
Flagella	Tail-like structure that helps control movement.
Pili	Hair-like projections that help bacteria attach to different surfaces, such as cells.
Facultative aerobic	Organism that prefers an environment without oxygen but has adapted to survive in the presence of oxygen. Examples include *Staphylococcus* spp. and *Lactobacillus.*
Microaerophilic aerobe	Organism that needs lower levels of oxygen than that typically found in the environment to survive and may also require higher levels of carbon dioxide. Examples include *Campylobacter* spp. and *Helicobacter pylori.*
Aerobic	Organism that lives and reproduces in an environment with oxygen. Obligate aerobes can only live in oxygenated environments. Example includes *Pseudomonas aeruginosa.*

| Facultative anaerobic | Organism that is able to live and reproduce in an environment with or without oxygen. Examples include *Escherichia coli* and *Streptococcus* spp. |
| Anaerobic | Organism that lives and reproduces in an environment without oxygen. Obligate anaerobes can only live in the absence of oxygen. Example includes *Clostridium botulinum.* |

MICROCONIDIA, MACROCONIDIA, ARTHROCONIDIA, AND BLASTOCONIDIA

1. Microconidia: Microconidia are spores that are produced by the asexual reproduction of a fungus (a conidophore). Microconidia are the smallest of the spores that are produced, and they are non-motile.
2. Macroconidia: Macroconidia are spores that are produced by the asexual reproduction of a fungus (a conidophore). The Macroconidia are the largest of the spores that are produced. They are non-motile.
3. Arthroconidia: Arthroconidia are spores that are created when fungal hyphae undergo segmentation. These spores are not very environmentally durable, and they are asexual in nature.
4. Blastoconidia: Blastoconidia are spores that are created when yeast cells undergo budding. They are also created through asexual reproduction.

BACTERIOSTATIC

A drug that is bacteriostatic is one that limits the reproduction and growth of new bacteria. Bacteriostatic antibiotics can do this by negatively affecting the cellular metabolism of bacteria. They also can hamper the production of the bacteria's DNA and protein. All of these interferences by the bacteriostatic drug have an effect on the growth and development of new bacteria. Some examples of bacteriostatic antibiotics are: Lincosamides, sulphonamides, tetracycline, and macrolides. Bacteriostatic antibiotics should be distinguished from bactericidal antibiotics, in that bactericidal antibiotics actually kill bacteria, whereas bacteriostatic antibiotics only curtail their reproduction. An example of bactericidal antibiotic is penicillin.

MYCOBACTERIUM

Bacteria belonging to the genus *Mycobacterium* are aerobic, non-motile, rod shaped bacteria. They have cell walls that are very thick and that contain a high quantity of lipids. This thick cell wall makes these bacteria hardy and resistant to acids, alcohol, some antibiotics, alkali solutions, dehydration, lysis, and some germicides. This can make infections caused by mycobacteria hard to treat. These bacteria can be either fast-growing or slow-growing, and because of this, they can be hard to culture in the laboratory. Mycobacteria are the cause of both tuberculosis and leprosy. In the laboratory, the presence of mycobacteria can be determined by an acid-fast stain, such as the Ziehl-Neelson stain.

MACCONKEY AGAR

MacConkey agar is a medium used in the laboratory to grow mycobacteria, such as *Mycobacteria chelonei*, and to differentiate between different types of mycobacteria. It is also used to stain gram negative bacteria for lactose fermentation. MacConkey agar consists of lactose, peptone, bile salts, crystal violet dye, and a neutral red dye. The red dye is what stains the bacteria that are fermenting the lactose present in the agar. MacConkey agar is used to not only identify various fast-growing mycobacteria, but it can be used to identify other pathogens, such as *Salmonella* and *Shigella*.

BACTERIAL CULTURE METHODS

DIFFERENT MEDIA

A number of different **media** are utilized for bacterial cultures, which are used to increase the numbers of a microorganism, select specific types, or differentiate them:

- Differential: The media changes in appearance with color change as a biochemical reaction to different bacteria, helping to distinguish different organisms.
- Selective: The media encourages the growth of one type of microorganism while inhibiting the growth of others.
- Enrichment: Media enriched with additives (such as sheep's blood) that encourages the growth of a specific type of microorganism.
- Candle jar: Inoculated specimen plates are placed inside of a glass jar and a small candle placed on top of the upper plate. As the candle burns, it uses up most of the oxygen and the carbon dioxide stimulates anaerobic bacterial growth although some aerobic growth may also occur because of residual oxygen.
- Living host cells: Used for some specific types of microorganisms that only grow in living cells, such as some leprosy.

ANAEROBIC MEDIA

Anaerobic microorganisms are most often found in abscesses and deep wounds, such as bites, blood, and cerebrospinal fluid. Aseptic technique is especially important to avoid contamination, and cotton swabs should not be used to collect a specimen because they may damage the microorganisms. Sample must be transported in an oxygen-free container.

- Anaerobic media: Pre-reduced anaerobically sterilized (PRAS) media is available, but is expensive and other media (selective, differential, or enriched) may be utilized as well if processed properly.
- Anaerobic techniques: Inoculated specimen plates are placed inside an anaerobic jar with an inlet and outlet and an electrified catalyst combines hydrogen and oxygen to provide anaerobic environment. With the gas pack, the inoculated plates are placed inside a container and water added combine hydrogen and oxygen, producing an anaerobic environment. Methylene blue is utilized as an anaerobic indicator.

ADDITIVES USED IN MEDIA PREPARATION

Media for culture must allow microorganisms to grow and reproduce, so various **additives** (nutrients or inhibitors) are added to an aqueous base to create different types of media. Complex media, which usually contain glucose and animal or plant proteins (protein hydrolysates such as tryptone), support various types of heterotrophic microorganisms. Defined media have exact percentages of various additives (such as mineral salts, growth factors, and simple carbohydrate) and support specific microorganisms and are generally required for microbiological assays. Selective media often have additives (such as mannitol) to suppress growth of undesirable microorganisms while promoting growth of others (such as *Staphylococcus aureus)*. Differential media have additives that help to distinguish different types of colonies. Enriched media contains additives (such as sheep blood or heated blood [chocolate]) to encourage increased growth of specific microorganisms. Commonly used additives include arginine, biotin, dextrin, galactose, glucose, lactose, mannitol, citric acid, sorbitol, and EDTA.

ANTIMICROBIAL AGENT EXAMPLES

1. Gentamicin works by interfering with protein synthesis. Gentamicin can be used to treat urinary tract infections.
2. Vancomycin works by interfering with the synthesis of bacterial cell walls. Vancomycin can be used to treat serious respiratory infections in patients that are allergic to penicillins.
3. Clindamycin works by interfering with protein synthesis. Clindamycin can be used to treat respiratory infections.
4. Rifampin works by interfering with the synthesis of bacterial ribonucleic acid (RNA). Rifampin is used to treat tuberculosis.
5. Penicillin works by interfering with the synthesis of bacterial cell walls. Penicillin can be used to treat pneumonia.
6. Tetracycline works by interfering with the synthesis of bacterial RNA. It can be used to treat infections of the respiratory tract.

SPECIMEN COLLECTION, PREPARATION, AND REJECTION CRITERIA

Specimens must be obtained following established protocols and in the proper tube or container with the correct additive, such as sodium citrate in a blood specimen. The specimen must be stored and/or transported in a manner appropriate to the type of specimen. **Rejection criteria** may vary according to the type of specimen and test, and specimens are generally not discarded until the ordering healthcare provider is notified. Rejection criteria may include:

- Incorrect tube or container.
- Incorrect or missing requisition/order.
- Specimen size insufficient for testing.
- Hemolysis evident.
- Specimen not correctly labeled.
- Tube/container leaking or contaminated with body fluids. (Note: critical specimens may be salvaged after tube/container thoroughly cleansed with 10% hypochlorite [bleach] solution.)
- Specimen contained in syringe with attached needle.
- Date/Collection time not noted on specimen.
- Specimen too old for testing.
- Specimen improperly stored/transported.

STAINING FLAGELLA TECHNIQUE

The most common technique used in the laboratory for the staining of flagella is the Leifson staining technique. Tannic acid-base fuchsin solution is used to stain the flagella that make bacteria mobile. The stain precipitates out along the filaments of the flagella, and the diameter of the flagella is increased. This then allows for the flagella to be easily visualized using light microscopy. The technique needs to be performed with care, however, to achieve accurate results Various aspects of the test need to be checked, such as the cleanliness of the glass slides used, the pH of the stain used, and the actual time the specimen spends submerged in stain.

CULTURING CLINICAL SPECIMENS

Blood	Obtain two (anaerobic and aerobic) 8-10 mL specimens at temperature peak and/or multiple at 30-minute to 1-hour intervals and inoculate the blood culture vials. Incubate and monitor as per protocol. Gram stain samples from positive cultures and subculture for aerobic (sheep blood, chocolate agar) and anaerobic organisms according to protocol (usually after 18-48 hours). Incubate at 35°-37°C for up to 7 days and inspect at least 2 times daily.
Urine	Obtain clean catch or catheterized specimen in sterile container. Process immediately or store specimen at 4°C. Prepare a slide for gram staining with one drop of mixed (not centrifuged) urine and examine under microscope or conduct the leukocyte esterase strip test. Negative findings generally indicate culture is unnecessary, but positive findings should be followed by inoculation of a MacConkey agar plate with incubation at 35°-37°C for 24-48 hours.
Stool	Collect specimen prior to beginning antibiotics in a sterile container or use cotton-tipped swab inserted into the rectum and rotated to obtain a fecal sample. Insert swab into sterile tube. The specimen should be processed as soon as possible or stored at 4°C. Specimen should be examined microscopically and plates inoculated. A fecal suspension with saline may be necessary for swabs or solid stool specimens if multiple plates must be inoculated. This also helps eliminate organic matter. Various types of agar may be used depending on the suspected organisms. Incubate at 35°-37°C for 24-48 hours.
Sputum	Collect sputum specimen in wide-mouthed sterile container and process within one hour. Record macroscopic appearance and prepare a gram-stain for microscopic examination. If fewer than 10 PMNs are noted per epithelial cells, the specimen should be rejected. If more, agar plates (various types) should be inoculated and incubated 35°-37°C for 24-48 hours (inspect after 18 hours).
Throat (upper respiratory)	Collect 2 specimens with sterile swabs rubbed over the back of the throat and tonsillar areas, avoiding the tongue and other structures, and place in sterile tube for transfer. Process within 4 hours or place in transport medium. Gram-staining is generally done only on specific request. Inoculate a blood agar (low glucose) by rubbing the swab over 1 quadrant and streak the remaining quadrants with a sterile loop. Place a bacitracin disk and a co-trimoxazole disk over the streaked area to aid in identification of bacteria. Incubate at 35°-37°C for 18 hours and inspect for colonies and then inspect again at 48 hours. Gram-stain colony samples to aid in identification.
Cerebrospinal fluid	Collect 5 to 10 mL CSF in 2 sterile tubes and process immediately. The CSF should be assessed macroscopically and microscopically through direct microscopy, gram-stain, and acid-fast stain. Inoculate plates appropriate to bacteria identified through microscopy or multiple media if unclear and incubate for at least 3 days with temperature and conditions determined by the type of agar and environment required for suspected organisms (aerobic, anaerobic).

Wound	Collect specimen through aspiration (preferred) of exudate or tissue sample or by wiping the wound with 2 cotton swabs and placing swabs in sterile container, in transport medium if processing cannot be done immediately. The exudate should be examined with direct, Gram-stain, and acid-fast stain microscopy and macroscopically (color, consistency, odor). Depending on results of the microscopic examination, various types of plates (minimum 3) should be inoculated. If using a swab for inoculation, wipe the swab across one quadrant of a plate and streak the remaining quadrants with a wire loop. Incubation time, temperature, and environment depend on the type of plate and the suspected organisms.
Abscess	Similar to wound culture although aspirant only is generally used. Organisms may be polymicrobial, including both aerobic and anaerobic bacteria, depending on the site of the abscess. Culturing for anaerobic bacteria (both gram-negative and gram-positive) should always be included, so the specimen must be protected from exposure to oxygen and incubation done at 35°C for 48 hours and then examined.
Genital fluids	<u>Females</u>: Collect specimen with pelvic examination and speculum moistened only with water. Wipe away mucus about the cervix with a cotton swab/ball and discard. Then insert a cotton swab and wipe the vaginal posterior fornix for the first sample, use another swab to collect an endocervical sample by inserting the swab into the cervix and rotating it for 10 seconds. <u>Males</u>: Collect oropharyngeal, urethral, anorectal specimens in a similar manner, inserting swab 3 to 4 cm inside urethra and 4 to 5 cm inside anus/rectum. <u>Examination</u>: Examine macroscopically for color and odor and through direct and gram-stain microscopy. Culturing should be done to identify *Neisseria gonorrhoeae* (especially in females) with direct inoculation of Thayer-Martin agar incubated at 35°C in candle-jar environment for 48 hours (checked daily for colonies).
Ear exudates	Collect specimens with two swabs inserted gently into the ear canal and rotated. Examine through direct and Gram-stain microscopy. Culture is usually carried out on MacConkey medium, blood agar, and Sabouraud dextrose medium with antibiotics, depending on the type of bacteria observed through microscopy with temperature and environment also dependent on suspected bacteria.
Eye exudate	Collect 2 specimens with a sterile cotton swab from the lower conjunctival sac and from the inner canthus of each eye and place in sterile tubes. Examine (first swabs) through direct, Gram-stain, and Giemsa stain microscopically and then carry out cultures (second swabs). Volume of bacteria for both ear and eye exudates tends to be low, so antibiotic disks are generally not used. Media commonly used includes MacConkey agar (under aerobic condition), blood agar (candle jar), and chocolate agar (candle jar). Incubate 18-24 hours, examine, and incubate another 48 hours if necessary.
Tissue	Collect specimens through surgical procedure or endoscopy and place in sterile container in transport medium. Examine macroscopically and microscopically. Process the tissue sample as per protocol for type of tissue and inoculate various types of culture media, depending on the tissue type and suspected microorganisms. Incubate at 35 to 37°C for times indicated for media.

IV catheter tips	Collect the IV catheter intact and transport in sterile container. Cut a 5 cm section from the catheter tip and roll that four times over a solid medium plate or immerse the section in broth culture medium. Incubate at 35° to 37°C for the times indicated for media and examine for colonies (>15 significant). Various other methods may be utilized, and blood cultures are usually done simultaneously.
IUD	Similar to procedures for IV catheter tips. Endocervical (and sometimes blood) cultures are usually done simultaneously.

ISOLATING, IDENTIFYING, AND DIFFERENTIATING MICROORGANISMS

Isolating, identifying, and differentiating microorganisms begin with direct examination under a microscope so that the shape, size, cell wall characteristics, and linkages can be noted. This helps to identify the basic type: bacilli, cocci, coccobacilli, and spirals. This is followed by Gram-staining, which helps to differentiate Gram-positive and Gram-negative organisms. Based on these assessments and suspected organism, various media are selected for culturing of the sample because some encourage the growth of certain organisms and others inhibit growth. The cultured plates are incubated to encourage growth of colonies and the colonies examined (size, shape, surface, texture, color) to further identify the organism. In some cases, sub-cultures are required to differentiate species. Additional methods include API® (test strips), biochemical testing, and carbohydrate fermentation tests. If the organism is still not identified, then DNA sequencing may be carried out.

PROCESSING AND PLANTING OF SPECIMENS
OBTAINING INOCULUM FROM AGAR AND BROTH

Processing and planting of specimens: Media used for cultures must be sterilized and maintained in sterile conditions and organisms transferred to the media using aseptic transfer techniques. Tube caps are removed and tops heated (up draft) to keep contamination away from the inside. Inoculation is typically made with a sterile inoculating needle (agar deeps) or wire loop (agar plates/broths). The inoculating needle or wire loop must be heated to red hot and cooled before transfer. To obtain inoculum:

- Agar plate: Lift one side of the lid (do not completely uncover) and use the wire loop to lift one colony (or part of a large colony) of the surface.
- Agar slant: Use the wire loop to scrape inoculum from the surface.
- Broth: Mix by shaking slightly and then immerse the loop and withdraw carefully (a film should be noted across the loop).

Note: For agar deep, obtain inoculum with a sterile needle.

INOCULATING AGAR AND BROTH

Processing and planting of specimens: Always maintain aseptic technique. To inoculate:

- Agar deep: Insert the needle straight to the bottom and withdraw straight.
- Agar plate: Lift one side of the lid and slide the loop in horizontally, streaking the inoculum back and forth on the surface only. Reflame the loop after each third of the plate is streaked, reinoculate, turn the plate 90° and continue until the entire plate (or 3 quadrants) is streaked. Invert plate for incubation.

- Agar slant: Either insert loop to the bottom of the tube and withdraw straight (for growth pattern) or in back-and-forth manner (for increased growth).
- Broth: Swish the loop back and forth about the tube.

Once inoculation is complete, then the plate/tube is placed in the incubator with the temperature and duration determined by the type of medium and the type of organism.

INTERPRETING/IDENTIFYING STRUCTURES THROUGH MICROBIOLOGICAL SLIDE PREPARATIONS

Direct (wet mount)	Because the organism is not fixed, motile organisms (such as *Vibrio)* and fragile organisms (such as those with filaments or sporulating bodies) are more easily identified. Wet mount is used for fecal examination for O & P. <u>Dark-field microscopy</u> helps to identify spirochetes, and <u>India ink preparation</u>, *C. neoformans.*
Direct (dry mount)	The organisms are killed, hardened, and adhered to the slide so they can't change shape or configuration. <u>Simple staining </u>(crystal violet, methylene blue [most commonly used], safranin, carbol-fuchsin) helps to identify gross morphology and to differentiate types of organisms. <u>Gram-staining</u> helps to differentiate Gram-positive from Gram-negative pathogens. Gram-staining also helps to determine the type of biochemical tests or culture media to use. <u>Acid fast staining</u> is used primarily to identify *Mycobacterium tuberculosis* and *M. leprae.* <u>Ziehl-Neelsen hot staining</u> utilizes carbol-fuchsin solution to diagnose *M. tuberculosis* from sputum sample.

NORMAL FLORA

Normal flora are those bacteria (predominate), fungi, and protists that are normally found on the surface tissues, including the skin and the mucous membranes. The most common bacteria are *Staphylococcus epidermidis* and *Staphylococcus aureus*, which are found on both skin and mucous membranes, as is *Streptococcus pyogenes.* Overgrowth of these organisms often results in skin infections, and these bacteria may migrate through open wounds. *Staphylococcus aureus* is a leading cause of infectious diseases. *Streptococcus mitis, salivarius, mutans, pneumoniae,* and *faecalis* are found on mucous membranes but not on the skin. Some bacteria are more common in one area of the body than others. For example, *Escherichia coli* is most common in the lower gastrointestinal tract, so it spreads through the fecal-oral route, and *Neisseria meningitidis* is found in the nose and pharynx, which allows it to spread through droplets.

RECOGNIZING AND IDENTIFYING PATHOGENS FROM CULTURES

Pathogen identification from cultures involves assessing colony morphology. Colonies may be circular, filamentous, rhizoid, or irregular in shape and may have various types of elevation, including flat, raised/rounded, convex, pulvinate, cratered, and knobby (umbonate). The colony margins may also help to identify organisms and may be solid, undulating, lobular/lobate, curled, or filamentous. The surface of the colony may vary according to the organism. Surfaces may, for example, be smooth, rough, granular, or glistening. The texture of the colony may range from dry or brittle to moist or viscous. The color of the colony may vary also depending on the medium and the organism. For example, on MacConkey agar, *Escherichia coli* colonies are pink. Colors may range from colorless, pink, red, blue, green, to black. The diameter (in millimeters) of the colonies varies according to the types of organism, so measuring the colonies can aid in identification.

SHAPES, ARRANGEMENTS, AND GROWTH CURVES OF BACTERIA

Cocci (spheres)	Single, in pairs (diplococci) (*Streptococcus pneumonia, Neisseria gonorrhoeae*), chains (*Streptococcus pyogenes*), tetrads (clusters of 4) (*Micrococcus sp.*), cubes (8 cocci) (*Sarcina*), or grapelike clusters (*Staphylococcus aureus*).
Bacilli (rods)	Single, in pairs (diplobacilli), chains (streptobacilli), or oval (coccobacilli). May be Gram-positive (*Clostridium, Listeria*) or gram-negative (*Enterobacter, Escherichia, Pseudomonas*).
Filamentous (thread-like)	Various shapes of bacteria can, under some conditions, form long chains and develop into filamentous bacteria, which may be straight or curved (*Sphaerotilus natans, Haliscomenobacter hydrossis*).
Spirochetes (spirals)	Single gram-negative bacteria (*Treponema pallidum, Borrelia burgdorferi*)
Growth curve	Microbial growth curve: <u>Lag phase</u> (zero growth during which cells are depleted and adapt to environment), <u>exponential phase</u> (new cell material synthesized and mass increased at constant rate until growth slows because of lack of nutrients or accumulation of toxins), <u>maximum stationary phase</u> (growth ceases and cell turnover [death of old cells and formation of new] occurs), and <u>decline phase</u> (death rate increases until it reaches a steady state until most cells have died, at which point the death rate slows, and a small number of survivors may remain).

SYSTEMS OF BACTERIAL IDENTIFICATION

Various systems of **bacterial identification** are utilized:

- <u>API</u>: Test strips with up to 20 biochemical tests provide 2- to 72-hour (depending on type of organism) identification of gram-negative, gram-positive, anaerobic, and yeast organisms, as well as strips for specific tests (such as carbohydrate metabolism) and organisms (such as *Lactobacillus* and *Bacillus*).
- <u>Automated</u>: Software is available for PCR and microarray-based identification systems.
- <u>Biochemical</u>: Organisms are identified by adding reagents to a substrate, which results in an enzymatic reaction that causes a color change that can be quantified. Different reagents are utilized to identify specific organisms. For example, TDA reagent is used to identify *Proteus* species.
- <u>Carbohydrate metabolism</u> (includes lactose fermentation, sucrose fermentation, glucose fermentation): This method identifies organisms by their ability ferment the carbohydrate. Broth containing lactose, sucrose, or glucose is inoculated with the suspected organism and a color change indicates fermentation is occurring. For example, the glucose fermentation can differentiate different species of *Enterobacteriaceae*.

AGAR DIFFUSION TESTING

Agar diffusion testing determines the antimicrobial effectiveness of a chemical. Streak a bacteria sample onto a nutrient-rich agar plate. The bacteria must be uniformly distributed on the plate, and Mueller-Hinton agar is the preferred agar for this analysis. Pipette various chemicals that are being tested onto numbered paper disks. Place these paper disks onto the streaked agar plate. Incubate at 37°C. Chemicals leach from the paper disks and spread outward onto the agar plate. Bacterial growth is not as prevalent in a clear ring surrounding a paper disk, so the chemical on that disk has antimicrobial effectiveness. Measure the clear areas (zones of inhibition) and compare the ring size to a standard atlas of zones of inhibition. The widest ring shows the most effective chemical.

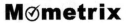

DILUTION TEST

The tube dilution test determines if chemicals being tested are either bactericidal or bacteriostatic in nature. Chemicals that are bactericidal are those that kill bacteria, while chemicals that are bacteriostatic do not kill bacteria, rather they inhibit the growth and reproduction of bacteria. Place a bacteria specimen in a tube, along with the particular chemical that is being tested. Place this mixture onto a nutrient-rich agar plate. If the bacteria are able to grow on the plate at all, then the chemical that is being tested is likely to have some bacteriostatic properties, since the bacteria were not killed. However, if no bacteria grow on the nutrient-rich agar plate, the bacteria must have been killed by the chemical being tested, which would make that chemical bactericidal.

TESTING FOR MULTI-DRUG RESISTANT TUBERCULOSIS (MDR-TB)

Testing for **multi-drug-resistant tuberculosis** (*Mycobacterium tuberculosis*) includes:

- Agar proportion: Use Felsin quadrant plates, which contain an antibiotic-impregnated disk in 3 quadrants with the remaining quadrant serving as the control. Molten Middlebrook 7H11 agar medium is poured over the antimicrobial disks and incubated overnight to allow the antibiotic agent to diffuse through the medium. Then each quarter is inoculated and the plate sealed and incubated at 37° C for 3 to 4 weeks. The organism is susceptible to the antibiotic if there is >200 colonies in the control quadrant and none in the antibiotic-containing quadrant.
- 96 well microtiter plate (MYCOTB): This method requires first growing colonies of the microorganism and then inoculating the wells in the microtiter plate. The plate contains 12 antimicrobial drugs in different concentrations (isoniazid, rifampin, ethambutol, kanamycin, cycloserine, amikacin, moxifloxacin, ofloxacin, rifabutin, streptomycin, ethionamide, and para-aminosalicylic acid. (Note pyrazinamide must be tested for separately because it requires an acidic environment). The plate is incubated for 14 days and the growth in each well is evaluated utilizing a mirror box or a semi-automatic plate reader.

OXIDASE TEST

The oxidase test is used to distinguish bacteria on the basis of whether they contain cytochrome c oxidase by using disks that contain a reagent that changes color when oxidized. Moisten each disk containing the reagent with de-ionized water. Place a sample of the bacteria on each disk with the reagent. After three minutes, observe the color of the disks. If there has been a color change to either maroon, blue, or black, then the reagent has been oxidized, and the bacteria is oxidase positive, or OX+. Oxidase positive bacteria can use oxygen for energy production, and they do contain cytochrome c oxidase. The Pseudomonadaceae are oxidase positive. If there is no color change after three minutes, then the reagent is reduced and the bacteria are oxidase negative (OX-). The Enterobacteriaceae are oxidase negative.

NAGLER TEST

The Nagler test is used to identify bacterial organisms that can produce lecithinases (phospholipases). One example of such an organism is *Clostridium perfringens*. Place the sample in question on an agar medium containing egg yolk. On one half of the agar medium, add the antitoxin for *Clostridium perfringens* type A. After incubation, a positive Nagler test will show the half of the test plate that contains the antitoxin is clear and has no evidence of lecithinase production. The half of the test plate that did not contain the antitoxin will show evidence of the production of lecithinase as an opaque area surrounding the bacterial sample.

NIACIN TEST

The niacin test is used to identify the presence of a specific type of mycobacteria, *Mycobacterium tuberculosis*. This particular mycobacterium releases a large quantity of niacin (B_3) during its metabolic processes. All mycobacteria release a certain amount of niacin, but only Mycobacterium tuberculosis releases enough to be of use in the niacin test. Culture the sample on egg based media for a three to four week incubation period before niacin testing. Add a cyanogen bromide (CNBr) solution and an aniline solution to the egg based bacterial culture. If niacin is present, a color change to yellow will be seen. If there is no color change, then *Mycobacterium tuberculosis* is not present. Care should be taken when performing the niacin test because cyanogen bromide solution is highly toxic. Wear a respirator, gloves, and use a fume hood.

INDOLE TEST

The indole test is performed on bacteria to determine its ability to produce indole from the degradation of tryptophan. Incubate a bacterial culture in a peptone or tryptophan broth for a 24 to 48 hour period. After this incubation period, add Kovac's reagent or Ehrlich's reagent to the broth and bacterial culture mixture. If the surface layer of the broth changes to red-violet or red in color, then the test is positive. An example of a bacterium that will have a positive result is *E. coli*. If the surface layer is yellow, however, the test is negative. *Salmonella* results in a negative indole test. A third result is possible, and that is if the surface layer of the broth turns orange. This is called a variable result. The variable result is due to presence of methyl indole, instead of indole.

BACTERIAL DIFFERENTIATING TESTS

Optochin susceptibility test utilizes disks (P) that contain optochin, to which *S. pneumoniae* are susceptible. The disk is placed on top of a blood agar plate covering zone one (area that is heavily inoculated with a specimen) and incubated. If growth is inhibited about the disk, this is an indication that the bacteria are *S. pneumoniae*.

Camp test is used to identify group B strep (particularly *Streptococcus agalactiae)* and gram-positive rods, which produces CAMP factor (extracellular protein) that acts in conjunction with beta-lysin (produced by *Staphylococcus aureus)* to promote hemolysis of sheep RBCs. The test utilizes a sheep blood agar plate, which is inoculated in a line across the plate with *Staphylococcus aureus.* The plate is then inoculated with the test specimen in a straight line perpendicular (2-3 cm in length) to the *Staph* line (at least 1 cm away and not touching it), placed in incubator at 37°C for 24-28 hours, and then checked to see if hemolysis has occurred from the interaction.

Indole test is used to differentiate Enterobacteriaceae genera (*Escherichia, Proteus, Salmonella, Shigella, Enterobacter)*, which are gram-negative facultative anaerobes that can break down tryptophan into indole. A 4-mL tube of tryptophan broth is inoculated with a sample from an 18-24 hour culture. The inoculated tube is then incubated at 37°C for 24-28 hours. Then 0.5 mL of Kovac's reagent is added to the tube and the color observed. If the sample is positive, a rose to bright red color change will appear in the top reagent layer. **Indole spot test** is used to differentiate indole positive members of a species from indole negative (such as *Klebsiella* pneumoniae (negative) from other *Klebsiella* spp. (positive). A few drops of Indole Spot reagent are placed on filter paper, which is inoculated with a sample of an 18-24 hour culture by rubbing the sample over the wet area of the paper. A color change occurs within 3 minutes: blue for positive and pink for negative.

Beta-lactamase (Cefinase) test (discs impregnated with Nitrocefin) is used to identify organisms (anaerobic bacteria, *Staphylococci, Enterococci, N. gonorrhoeae,* and *Haemophilus influenzae,* which produce beta-lactamase. One sample is used for each disk. Place disks on empty Petri dish and place one drop of sterile distilled water on each disk. Inoculate disks with colonies and note change in disk color to yellow or red for positive organisms. Time to reaction varies according to organism:

- 1 minute: H. influenzae, N. gonorrhoeae.
- 5 minutes: Enterococcus faecalis.
- 30 minutes: Anaerobic bacteria.
- 60 minutes: Staphylococcus aureus.

Oxidase test is used to identify aerobic bacteria that produce cytochrome oxidase (an enzyme). A small sample of the organism culture is removed from an agar plate or slant tube (being careful not to include any agar) with a swab and one drop of reagent used to dampen the culture. If the bacteria are aerobic, a positive reaction will cause the dampened swab/culture to turn violet to purple in 10-30 seconds.

Catalase test is used to identify aerobic organisms (*Staphylococcus*), which are usually catalase positive and can release oxygen from hydrogen peroxide, resulting in production of a white froth. This test should not be done on blood agar but rather on samples in slant tubes after 18-24 hours of growth. A few drops of hydrogen peroxide are added to the slant tube and observed for froth reaction. If the results appear negative, a sample can be placed under a microscope and the hydrogen peroxide added to more easily observe the reaction.

Tryptic soy broth (TSB) with NaCl (6.5%) is used to assess whether an organism can live in a high-salt environment. While most organisms die, *Enterococci, Aerococci,* and *Staphylococci* can tolerate the environment and continue to grow. Tubes with TSB with NaCl (6.5%) are inoculated with a bacterial sample and incubated at 37°C. A positive finding occurs if the solution becomes cloudy from the growth of organisms.

Mannitol salt agar test contains mannitol (10 g), a sugar; beef extract (1 g); proteose peptone #3 (10 g); NaCl 75 g, agar (15 g), phenol red (0.025 g), a pH indicator; and 1 distilled water (1000 mL). The solution is heated until clear, autoclaved at 121°C, cooled and poured into Petri dishes. The high salt concentration inhibits most bacteria, but *Staphylococcus* species are able to ferment the mannitol, and this produces an acid that changes the pH of the phenol and causes the agar to change from red to yellow.

Bacitracin disks contain 0.04 units of bacitracin, to which group A *Streptococcus* is susceptible. The disk is placed on top of a blood agar plate covering zone one (area that is heavily inoculated with a specimen) and incubated. If growth is inhibited about the disk, this is an indication of group A *Streptococcus.*

Bile solubility test is done to identify *S. pneumoniae.* A drop of 10% sodium deoxycholate is placed on top of an established suspected colony (after 18-24 hours of growth) and then incubated for 15-30 minutes at 37°C. If *S. pneumoniae* is present, this procedure will cause lysis of the cells.

Coagulase bile esculin (*Enterococcus* slant) test is done to identify *Enterococcus.* The medium contains beef extract (3 g), peptone (5 g), oxgall (40 g), esculin (0.5 g), ferric citrate (0.5 g), agar (15 g), and distilled water (1000 mL). The solutions is heated, pH adjust to 7.09, autoclaved at 121°C for 15 minutes, cooled to 55°C, and poured into sterile tubes and allowed to set with the tubes in slanted rather than upright position. (Note: Before filling tubes, 50 mL horse serum may be added to the solution, but this is optional). Once the agar has set, inoculate the slants with organisms from the primary plate. *Enterococcus,* which is esculin positive, will form brown-black colonies with a surrounding black zone.

STREPTOCOCCAL TESTING

Streptococcus infections include strep throat, scarlet fever, rheumatic fever, necrotizing fasciitis, urinary tract infections, psoriasis, and pneumonia.

Throat swabs: rapid enzyme immunoassay (more accurate for positives than negatives) (group A)	A number of different rapid strep kits are available that are able to detect strep group A. The tests usually begin with a tonsillar and throat swab. The swab is then swirled inside of a tube holding a mixture of 2 reagents, left in place for about 1 minute, and then removed and a test strip inserted, timed, and checked against a color chart. Antibody/antigen sensitivity tests also help to identify strep.
Beta-hemolytic strep (group B) screening for *S. agalactiae*.	Commonly colonizes in intestinal, urinary, and reproductive systems and can infect the fetus in late pregnancy, so screening of pregnant women is done routinely with rectal and vaginal cultures because most are asymptomatic. While the strep is not usually pathogenic to the mother, the newborn may develop pneumonia (newborns lack alveolar macrophages) or meningitis.
Bacterial identification	Streptococci are gram-positive cocci that occur in pairs or chains and are facultative anaerobes. Streptococci grow on blood agar, chocolate agar, and (some species) on PEA. Cultured colonies are small, gray, and slightly raised and appear translucent with a margin around the entire colony.
	Streptococci are catalase negative, esculin negative, MSA, and optochin negative, and these tests can differentiate strep from other cocci.
	Alpha-hemolytic strep (*S. pneumoniae*, which is optochin susceptible and bile soluble) exhibits only partial hemolysis.
	Beta-hemolytic strep includes group A strep (*S. pyogenes*, which exhibit strong beta-hemolysis and bacitracin inhibition) and group B strep (*S. agalactiae*, identified by the CAMP test). Beta-hemolytic strep cases complete hemolysis.

CLOSTRIDIUM DIFFICILE TOXIN TESTS

Clostridium difficile can release a toxin that can cause necrosis of the colon. A variety of tests are available to test stool for ***Clostridium difficile* toxin**, and the time needed may vary from a few hours to several days (more sensitive). The two-step procedure is recommended:

- Step 1: Glutamate dehydrogenase (GDH) test: This is a rapid screening test that shows if the *Clostridium difficile*-produced antigen, glutamate dehydrogenase, is present, but does not differentiate between strains that produce toxin and those that do not.
- Step 2 choices:
- Cell cytotoxicity culture (takes 24-48 hours): Tissue test that identifies the cytotoxin on tissue cells.

- Stool culture on fresh stool (takes 2-3 days): Can identify toxin but not cannot differentiate colonization from overgrowth of the organism, so further toxin testing, such as tests for toxin A and B, must be done. Testing should be done as soon as possible or sample refrigerated as toxins rapidly degrade.
- PCR assay: Results are available rapidly and test is sensitive but is expensive and not widely available.

CAMPYLOBACTER PYLORI SCREENING

Microscopic	Microorganism may be observed in the feces in a fresh specimen (≤2 hours) or from cultures.
Culture & Sensitivities	Microorganism is more difficult than other enteric microorganism to culture and requires use of special blood agar that contains antibiotics, micropore filtration, and incubation at 42°C.
ELISA	Antigen testing allows for serodiagnosis.
PCR	Able to directly detect the microorganism in stool.
Serology	Tests for presence of antibodies, but they may not be detected early in the infection so the test should be repeated within 10 to 14 days.
Rapid urease (RUT)	6% RUT most accurate and test results may be available within 10 minutes (compared to other microorganisms that show positive results after a longer period of time).

HELICOBACTER PYLORI SCREENING

Antigen	Fecal test often used for diagnosis. Positive if the *H. pylori* antigen or traces of the microorganism are detected.
Antibody	Serum test can identify antibodies to *H. pylori* but cannot differentiate previous infection from current, so not used for diagnosis and positive finding must be confirmed.
Urea breath	Solution containing urea is swallowed and level of carbon dioxide measured in exhaled breaths 10 minutes later as H. pylori converts urea to carbon dioxide.
Microscopic	Tissue sample (GI) may show presence of *H. pylori.*
Culture & sensitivities	Culture of *H. pylori* is generally done only if necessary susceptibility testing for antibiotics.
Rapid urease	The enzyme urease (produced by *H. pylori)* may be detected in tissue sample.
PCR	Generally not necessary for diagnosis but may be used for research purposes.

ANTIMICROBIAL SUSCEPTIBILITY TESTING

Antimicrobial susceptibility testing is done to determine which antibiotic an organism is susceptible to. The Kirby-Bauer test (disk diffusion test) is one method:

- Select 3 to 5 colonies and prepare with direct colony suspension or the log phase method.
- Inoculate a Mueller-Hinton agar plate (4 mm depth) or other medium specific to the organism.
- Apply antimicrobial disks individually or with automatic disk dispenser within 15 minutes of inoculation.

- Invert plate and incubate at required temperature and duration, generally between 16 and 24 hours.
- Measures zones of inhibition from the back of the plate, using reflected or transmitted light depending on the organism.

Many factors can affect the results of manual testing: incubation temperature and duration, type of medium, bacterial growth rate, depth of the medium, procedures for reading results. Automated systems generally provide more reliable results and have test panels available for specific organisms as well as gram-positive and gram-negative bacteria.

ANTIMICROBIAL SUSCEPTIBILITY TESTING

Minimum inhibitory concentration (MIC) testing is used to determine the lowest antimicrobial concentration that is effective in inhibiting growth of the organism. Commercial plates and panels are available. For example, the broth microdilution MIC test includes a panel with 96 wells (0.1 mL) for inoculation while the agar dilution MIC test includes agar medium plates with different antimicrobial concentrations; however, the MIC test with agar plates is time consuming and more difficult to quantify. Incubation duration varies from 16 to 24 hours, depending on the organism. The MIC endpoint is the concentration at which growth is completely inhibited or >80% compared to the control for some antibiotics. Automated systems are available for antimicrobial susceptibility testing. For example, a well card may be automatically incubated and read by a photometer and the MIC calculated by a computerized program.

GRAM'S METHOD OF STAINING BACTERIA

Gram staining method is used to distinguish between gram-positive and gram-negative bacteria in the laboratory. Stain the sample with crystal violet. Next, treat the sample with a solution of iodine. Add alcohol or another organic solvent to the sample. Examine the sample under the microscope. Gram-positive bacteria will still be stained a violet/blue color. Gram-negative bacteria, however, will be colorless. In order to make the gram-negative bacteria stand out, counterstain the sample with safrinin. This counterstain will make the gram-negative bacteria appear red in color, and the gram-positive bacteria will still appear violet/blue in color.

GRAM-POSITIVE BACTERIA VS. GRAM NEGATIVE BACTERIA STAIN RETENTION

In the Gram test, gram-positive bacteria will retain their bluish/violet color from the crystal violet stain even after being treated with an organic solvent. Gram-negative bacteria, on the other hand, will lose their color and appear colorless after being treated with an organic solvent. Gram-negative bacteria have a very thin cell wall, so when they are washed with the alcohol, the stain is liberated from the bacteria. Gram-positive bacteria, on the other hand, have a very thick cell wall made of peptidoglycan, so the alcohol solvent is not able to liberate the violet stain from the bacteria.

USES OF VARIOUS STAINS IN THE LABORATORY

1. Crystal violet is used for the gram staining of bacterial cell walls. Gram-negative bacteria will appear red or pink in color, and gram-positive bacteria will appear dark blue or violet in color when treated with crystal violet.
2. Wright's stain is used to help distinguish blood cells. It can be used with either blood or bone marrow samples. Often it is used when performing white blood cell (WBC) counts if infections are expected in the patient.
3. Sudan black B is a stain that is used to identify the presence of triglycerides or lipids. Sudan black B will stain these compounds a bluish-black color.

4. Giemsa stain is a stain that can be used to identify bacteria and other parasites. Giemsa stain can be used with blood films, blood smears, or bone marrow samples. Giemsa stain will stain parasites or bacterial cells a purple color, while the human cells will be colored pink. Giemsa stain is made of a combination of eosin and methylene blue.

ISOLATING, IDENTIFYING, AND DIFFERENTIATING GRAM-POSITIVE COCCI

When gram-staining, gram-positive organisms stain purple and gram-negative organisms stain red ("Purple for positive"). Hemolysis may occur as a reaction on blood agar plates: Alpha (hemoglobin converts to form that appears shows as green, Beta (true hemolysis), and Gamma (nonhemoloytic).

Gram-positive cocci include:

Genera	Species	Differentiation
Staphylo-coccus (catalase positive and occur in clusters)	*S. aureus*	Beta/gamma hemolytic, positive for coagulase positive for mannitol fermentation, sensitive to novobiocin.
	S. epidermidis	Gamma hemolytic, negative for coagulase production, negative for mannitol fermentation, sensitive to novobiocin.
	S. saprophyticus	Same as *S. epidermidis* except resistant to novobiocin.
Strepto-coccus (catalase negative, grow in chains)	*S. pyogenes*	Lancefield group A, Beta hemolytic, sensitive to bacitracin (A disc).
	S. agalactiae	Lancefield group B, Beta or gamma hemolytic, positive CAMP tests
	S. pneumoniae	Non-groupable, Alpha hemolytic, bile soluble, sensitive to optochin (P disc).
Entero-coccus (catalase negative, similar to strep)	*E. faecalis*	Lancefield group D, Gamma hemolytic. Ferments mannitol and grows on mannitol salt agar
	E. faecium.	Lancefield group D, Gamma hemolytic. Does not ferment mannitol or grow on mannitol salt agar.

ISOLATING, IDENTIFYING, AND DIFFERENTIATING GRAM-POSITIVE BACILLI

Gram-positive bacilli (rod-shaped bacteria)

Genera	Species	Differentiation
Bacillus (spore producing)	*B. anthracis*	Associated with anthrax infection.
		Large cell, end-to-end chains, no motility, has poly-D-glutamic acid capsule.
	B. cereus	Associated with GI infections.
		Large cell, 50% of strains are motile.
Corynebacterium	*C. diphtheriae*	Associated with diphtheria.
		Small, narrow cell, no spores, no motility, pleomorphic, Chinese characters.
Listeria	*L. monocytogenes*	Associated with listeriosis, GI infection.
		Small cell. No spores, motility (tumbling), grow at 4°C intracellularly.

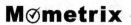

ISOLATING, IDENTIFYING, AND DIFFERENTIATING GRAM-NEGATIVE COCCI

GRAM-NEGATIVE COCCI

Genera	Species	Differentiation
Neisseria **(Diplococci)**	*N. gonorrhoeae*	Associated with sexually-transmitted disease.
		Positive oxidase, coffee-bean shaped, glucose positive, maltose negative, media—chocolate and Thayer-Martin agar.
	N. meningitidis	Associated with meningitis.
		Positive oxidase, kidney-bean shaped, glucose positive, maltose positive, media—blood or chocolate agar.
Moraxella **(Diplococcus)**	*M. catarrhalis*	Associated with respiratory infection.
		Positive oxidase, kidney-bean shaped, glucose negative, maltose negative, media—blood or chocolate agar.

ISOLATING, IDENTIFYING, AND DIFFERENTIATING GRAM-NEGATIVE COCCOBACILLI

GRAM-NEGATIVE COCCOBACILLI (RODS THAT ARE SHORT OR ROUND, SIMILAR TO COCCI)

Genera	Species	Differentiation
Haemophilus **(influenza)**	*H. influenzae*	Needs both factor X (hemin) and V (NAD) to grow. Cannot grow on blood agar but will grow about a streak line of β-hemolytic *Staphylococcus aureus* on blood agar (satellitism) because the *Staph* liberates factor. Media—Chocolate agar.
	H. ducreyi	Needs only factor X to grow. Media—Chocolate agar and rabbit blood agar.
Acinetobacter **(HA infections)**	*A. baumannii*	Standard ID not available. Differentiated by multiplex PCR OXA-51 typing.
Kingella **(Invasive infections)**	*K. Kingae*	In pairs or chains, often resistive to gram staining, beta-hemolytic, nonmotile, does not form spores. Negative catalase, negative urease, and negative indol tests but usually positive to oxidase.
Francisella **(Tularemia)**	*F. tularensis*	Non-motile, does not form spores. Media—Chocolate agar (enriched), buffered charcoal yeast extract. Culture often not successful, so ID is by DNA methods, immunoblotting, and antigen ELISA.

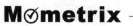

ISOLATING, IDENTIFYING, AND DIFFERENTIATING GRAM-NEGATIVE BACILLI

GRAM-NEGATIVE BACILLI (RODS)

Genera	Species	Differentiation
Bacteroides	*B. fragilis*	Rod-shaped, non-motile, negative oxidase, Negative H_2S gas, obligate anaerobic.
Campylobacter	*C. jejuni*	Comma, corkscrew, or S-shaped, motile, negative glucose fermentation, positive oxidase, negative lactose fermentation, negative H2S gas, and growth optimal at 42°C. Microaerophilic.
	C. coli	S-shaped. Similar to *C. jejuni*. Differentiated from *C. jejuni* by real-time assay.
	C. fetus	S-shaped, motile, microaerophilic, growth optimal on Butzler agar and CCDA agar, but no growth on MacConkey agar, catalase and oxidase positive, colistin-resistant.
Escherichia	*E. coli*	Rod-shaped, motile, positive glucose fermentation, negative oxidase, positive lactose fermentation, and negative H_2S gas.
Helicobacter	*H. pylori*	Spiral-shaped, motile, negative glucose fermentation, positive oxidase, negative lactose fermentation, and negative H_2S gas. Produces urease.
Salmonella	*S. enterica*	Rod-shaped, motile, positive glucose fermentation, Negative oxidase, negative lactose fermentation, and positive H_2S gas. Black on hektoen agar.
	S. typhi	Rod-shaped, facultative anaerobe, has H, O, and Vi antigens, catalase positive, oxidase and urease negative, vancomycin resistant, colistin susceptible. Black on hektoen agar.
Shigella	*S. flexneri*	Rod-shaped, nonmotile, positive glucose fermentation, negative oxidase, negative lactose fermentation, negative H_2S gas.
	S. dysenteriae	Rod-shaped, non-spore forming, facultative anaerobe, nonmotile, negative lactose fermentation and negative lysine. Green on hektoen agar.
Yersinia	*Y. enterocolitica*	Rod-shaped, nonmotile, positive glucose fermentation, negative oxidase, negative lactose fermentation, and negative H_2S gas.
Vibrio	*V. parahaemolyticus*	Comma-shaped, motile, facultative anaerobe, non-spore forming, positive glucose fermentation, positive glucose fermentation, negative lactose fermentation, negative H2S gas. Optimal growth in high salt environment.

Genera	Species	Differentiation
	V. vulnificus	Facultative anaerobe, non-spore forming, motile, curved or straight rods. Negative growth in 0% NaCl and positive in 1% NaCl. Positive lactose fermentation, positive oxidase, positive nitrate to nitrite, negative myo-inositol fermentation, negative arginine dihydrolase, positive lysine decarboxylase, 10%-89% positive ornithine decarboxylase.
	V. cholerae	Facultative anaerobe, non-spore forming, motile, positive growth in 0% and 1% NaCl, negative lactose fermentation, oxidase positive, positive nitrate to nitrite, negative myo-inositol fermentation, negative arginine dihydrolase, positive lysine decarboxylase and ornithine decarboxylase.

ENTEROBACTERIACEAE

Bacteria belonging to the family Enterobacteriaceae are gram-negative, anerobic, rod-shaped bacteria. They also produce lactic acid by fermenting sugars. Most of the Enterobacteriaceae are mobile, using flagella to move, but a few members are non-mobile. Bacteria from this family are normal flora in the guts and intestines of healthy humans, in soil or water, or in plants. Some are parasitic. Some examples of bacteria that belong to the family Enterobacteriaceae are *E. coli* and *Salmonella*.

DETERMINING IF ANEROBES ARE GRAM-POSITIVE OR GRAM-NEGATIVE EXAMPLES

1. Wolinella succinogens is gram-negative.
2. *Clostridium tetani* is gram-positive.
3. Bifidobacterium eriksonii is gram-positive.
4. *Veillonella* is gram-negative.
5. Lactobacillus catenaforme is gram-positive.

SPIROCHETES

Spirochetes are primitive bacteria that have a coiled or spiral shape that seem to pulsate under the microscope. These bacteria are gram-negative, and most are anerobic. Spirochetes contain flagella between their cell wall and the cell membrane, referred to as axial filaments, and they provide motility for the spirochetes. There are three families of spirochetes: *Leptospira*, *Borrelia burgdorferi*, and *Treponema pallidum*. Most spirochetes are pathogenic, causing diseases such as syphilis and Lyme disease. Spirochetes are also often found in liquid environments, and they can be transmitted to humans by organisms such as ticks and lice. In the laboratory, phase optics or dark-field optics or silver impregnation can be used to identify the presence of spirochetes.

Diseases caused by spirochetes and their transmission:

1. *Treponema pallidum pertenue* is the bacteria responsible for yaws. Yaws primarily affects children and is transmitted by flies.
2. *Treponema pallidum pallidum* is the bacteria responsible for syphilis. Syphilis is transmitted during sexual intercourse or from mother to child during pregnancy.
3. *Borrelia burgdorferi* is the bacteria responsible for Lyme disease. Lyme disease is transmitted from bites of infected deer ticks.

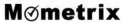

4. *Leptospira* is the bacteria responsible for leptospirosis. Leptospirosis can be transmitted from infected animals (such as cows or pigs) to humans or via infected soil or water.

5. *Treponema pallidum carateum* is the bacteria responsible for pinta. Pinta is often transmitted between children living in unsanitary conditions.

SYMPTOMS OF *SALMONELLA* FOOD POISONING

Salmonella in humans can be contracted by ingesting food, such as poultry, meat, or eggs, or drinking water that has been infected with *Salmonella*. Cutting boards that have come in contact with infected food transmit *Salmonella*. It is hard to know if a foodstuff or water is infected with *Salmonella* without laboratory tests being performed because it does not produce an "off" smell or taste. Therefore, humans will eat infected foods or water without knowing of the presence of *Salmonella*. Some symptoms of a *Salmonella* infection include fever, chills, nausea, stomach pain, excessive vomiting and diarrhea, and headache. The onset of symptoms can occur within six to seven hours from the time of *Salmonella* ingestion, or the onset of symptoms can take up to three days. Usually, *Salmonella* infection can be cured with antibiotic treatment.

TRENCH FEVER

Trench fever is an infection that is caused by *Rochalimaea quintana* and is transmitted to humans via a body louse, *Pediculus humanus*. The disease got its name from the many soldiers during World War I and World War II that contracted this disease. Today, it is most common in people who live in unsanitary conditions, such as the homeless. Some of the symptoms of trench fever are a fever, muscle and joint pain in the legs, headaches, chills, and a rash. The symptoms of the infection can last for long periods at a time, up to 2 weeks, and it can relapse as well. In the laboratory, the Weil-Felix test can identify the presence of *Rochalimaea quintana*. Treatment of trench fever is usually accomplished with tetracycline antibiotics.

ETIOLOGIC AGENTS ASSOCIATED WITH VARIOUS DISEASES

Disease	Associated Etiologic Agent
rabbit fever	*Francisella tularensis*
peptic ulcer disease	*Helicobacter pylori*
keratitis	*Pseudomonas aeruginosa*
whooping cough	*Bordetella pertussis*
Lyme disease	*Borrelia burgdorferi*
yaws	*Treponema pertenue*
scalded skin syndrome	*Staphylococcus aureus*
rat bite fever	*Streptobacillus moniliformis*
syphilis	*Treponema pallidum*
Weil's disease	*Leptospira*

NOCARDIACEAE

Bacteria in the family Nocardiaceae are aerobic, gram-positive, and rod-shaped. They are often found in organic rich soil, and they can cause pneumonia, cellulitis, and abscesses. Most often, people with compromised immune systems, the young, and the elderly are those that are affected by bacteria belonging to the Nocardiaceae. In the laboratory, these bacteria are able to grow in a wide range of temperatures, but they are slow growers when placed on non-selective culture media. They are partially acid fast and catalase-positive (bubbles form when Nocardiaceae are mixed with hydrogen peroxide in the catalase test).

MICROCOCCACEAE

The Micrococcaceae are spherical in shape, gram-positive, aerobic bacteria. They are catalase positive, forming bubbles when mixed with hydrogen peroxide in the catalase test. They are non-motile, and they can produce colored pigments (yellow, orange, or red). Some of the Micrococcaceae are harmless and others can cause disease. In fact, many Micrococcaceae are normal flora found on healthy human bodies. Two examples of Micrococcaceae are *Micrococcus* and *Staphylococcus*. These two bacteria look similar, but a way to tell them apart is that *Micrococcus* are oxidase positive, whereas *Staphylococcus* are oxidase negative.

BOTULISM

Botulism is an illness that is caused by *Clostridium botulinum*. This bacteria is gram-positive, anerobic, and spore-forming. There are seven serotypes of botulism, types A, B, C, D, E, F, and G. However, types A, B, E, and F are the only serotypes that cause illness in humans. Types A and B are most often due to botulism from ingesting canned foods, and type E is most often caused by eating fish that contain botulism spores. There are three main types of botulism that affect humans, and these are wound botulism, food borne botulism, and infant botulism (usually from babies less than 12 months old ingesting honey).

TYPES OF BOTULISM

Wound botulism is due to the release of toxins from Clostridium botulinum. This leads to various neurological symptoms in the affected person. **Food borne botulism** is due to the eating of foods that contain the toxin from *Clostridium botulinum*, like home canned foodstuffs. Food borne botulism can lead to neurological and gastrointestinal symptoms, as well as muscle weakness and fatigue. Food borne botulism can be mild or severe, depending on the amount of toxin ingested. **Infant botulism** is the most common form of botulism in the United States, and it occurs in young infants (only a few months old or younger). In this form of botulism, the infant eats a food that contains botulism spores, and the spores then grow in the infant's intestine, where they produce their toxin. This can lead to neurological and muscular problems, constipation, as well as the development of a "floppy head", which is characteristic of infant botulism.

TETANUS

Tetanus is a disease that is characterized the spastic contraction of voluntary muscles in the body. Muscles in the jaw and the neck are most often affected, hence the name, "lock jaw". This contraction of muscles can cause difficulty in breathing and/or convulsions in affected persons. The disease can be fatal if not treated quickly. Vaccinations can help prevent the development of tetanus. Tetanus is caused by a neurotoxin, tetanospasmin, which is produced by the anaerobic bacteria *Clostridium tetani* commonly found in dirt and soil, as well as in the intestines of humans and other animals. However, in the intestines, enzymes help destroy the tetanospasmin toxin, so this toxin in the intestines is not a health issue. Most people who do get infected with tetanus do so through open wounds or cuts, which get contaminated with *Clostridium tetani* present in dirt.

TOXIC SHOCK SYNDROME

Toxic shock syndrome (TSS) is a disease that is caused by a toxin producing strain of a common bacterium, *Staphylococcus aureus*. This toxin is called toxic shock syndrome toxin number 1, or TSST-1. Toxic shock syndrome was first reported in the 1970s in the United States, and it is most often seen in menstruating women who use tampons to control menstrual flow. However, TSS can be seen in debilitated patients, too. The incidence of toxic shock syndrome in the US has been declining because of changes in the composition of tampons on the market. Some symptoms of TSS include a high fever, diarrhea, a sunburn-like rash, muscle tenderness, and low blood pressure. If not treated immediately with antibiotics, shock or multiple organ failure/damage can develop. The disease can be fatal if not treated right away.

MOLECULAR ASSAYS IN BACTERIOLOGY

Molecular assays in bacteriology are able to identify bacteria or specific strains of bacteria based on their genetic sequences. Test results are usually available within hours rather than the days that may be required for cultures. A number of different tests are available:

- Direct PCR/gene sequencing: Sterile body fluid/tissue specimen used for amplification and sequencing. Isolates identified by sequencing of ribosomal RNA (purified DNA not necessary).
- Direct real time PCR for specific pathogens: Mycobacterium tuberculosis, Clostridium difficile, Bordetella pertussis, Bordetella parapertussis, Shiga-toxin producing Escherichia coli (including serotypes), Salmonella enterica, Shigella spp., group B Streptococcus agalactiae, Streptococcus pyogenes, and Streptococcus group C/G.
- PCR gene detection: MecA and BlaZ.
- Pulsed field gel electrophoresis strain typing: Used to identify different strains of organisms, such as *Staphylococcus aureus*.
- Multiplex PCR: Multiple targets are amplified in one PCR test.

REPRODUCTIVE METHODS OF VARIOUS PHYLA OF FUNGI

1. Chytridiomycota: Chytridiomycota experience asexual reproduction. This reproduction produces spores that have flagella and are motile in liquid environments. The spores that are produced are called zoospores.
2. Zygomycota: Zygomycota are terrestrial fungi, and they reproduce zygospores through sexual reproduction. An example of a fungus belonging to the phyla Zygomycota is black bread mold.
3. Glomeromycota: Glomeromycota produce blastophores through asexual reproduction. A single species has been noted, however, to produced zygospores through sexual reproduction.
4. Ascomycota: Ascomycota are referred to as sac fungi and they produce ascospores that are enclosed in a sac called an ascus. Their reproduction can be sexual or asexual, and the specific type of reproduction tends to vary. However, most produce through asexual measures.
5. Basidiomycota: Basidiomycota are known as the club fungi. They undergo sexual reproduction, producing basidiosphores. The basidiosphores are produced on basidi, which are club shaped stalks. Most mushrooms are part of this phyla.

KAUFFMAN-WHITE CLASSIFICATION SYSTEM

The Kauffman-White classification system is a system used to differentiate between the serologically different types of *Salmonellae*. This involves the determination of the surface antigens on the bacteria. The "O" (somatic) antigens are determined first. These antigens are polysaccharides, and they are associated with the outer membrane of the bacteria. The "H" (flagellar) antigens are determined next. They are proteins that are associated with the flagella on motile Salmonella found in the sample. Salmonella can be motile or non-motile. Determining which of the "O" and the "H" antigens are present can differentiate the salmonella.

DISEASES OR ILLNESSES ASSOCIATED WITH AEROBIC BACTERIA

1. *Mycobacterium tuberculosis* is the cause of tuberculosis.
2. *Pseudomonas aeruginosa* is the cause of swimmer's ear.

3. *Legionella pneumophila* is the cause of both legionnaires' disease and Pontiac fever.
4. *Bordetella pertussis* is the cause of whooping cough.
5. *Mycobacterium leprae* is the cause of leprosy.
6. *Chlamydia trachomatis* is the cause of trachoma.

ALPHA GROUP (A) AND BETA GROUP (B) STREPTOCOCCI

Alpha group streptococci are responsible for the majority of streptococcal disease in humans. Alpha group streptococci can cause scarlet fever, pneumonia, strep throat, and other upper respiratory infections. They also cause partial hemolysis of red blood cells. Beta group streptococci are also implicated in the hemolysis of red blood cells. They are referred to as hemolytic streptococci. Beta group strep is more harmful to red blood cells than streptococci of the alpha group. Beta strep can affect both white blood cells and the ability of blood to clot or agglutinate. Beta group strep is most harmful for newborn babies and kidney patients.

BETA GROUP STREP AND NEWBORNS

Beta group strep (hemolytic B strep) affects primarily newborn children. Newborns can catch beta group strep from their mothers either before or during birth. If a newborn becomes infected with group B strep, the baby can get very sick with meningitis or pneumonia. If left untreated, these infections can be fatal. In the United States, pregnant women are tested for group B strep during the third trimester of pregnancy, and if they are colonizers of the disease, they will be given an injection of antibiotics during labor to prevent the spread of group B strep to their babies. It is important to note that most adults who are colonizers of group B strep have no symptoms or adverse effects.

LYME DISEASE

Lyme disease is caused by the spirochete Borrelia burgdorferi. This disease is transmitted to humans and other animals (such as dogs and deer) via tick bites. It is not transmitted from human to human. After an infected tick has bitten a human, for example, the bacteria from the tick can enter the host through the skin. Most often, the body will be able to fight off the bacteria, but if not, it can remain in the skin of the host or it can spread through the bloodstream or the lymphatic system. It is possible for the bacteria to eventually spread to the central nervous system, the heart, or the joints of its host. There are three stages of Lyme disease, and each of these stages has certain symptoms associated with it. Early localized Lyme disease is characterized by flu-like symptoms and a possible rash called an erythema migrans. Early disseminated Lyme disease is characterized by arthritis-like pain, headaches, conjunctivitis, and continued fatigue. Finally, late-stage Lyme disease causes joint and neurological problems.

SEPTICEMIA

Septicemia (blood poisoning) is a disease that is caused by the spread of bacteria and/or their toxins throughout the blood stream. Septicemia is usually caused by the spread of gram-positive bacteria, usually staphylococci or streptococci and their released toxins. Localized infections (such as abscesses), various systemic diseases (such as meningitis), infections of tissues that are rapidly progressing, or infections of the blood vessel walls can all cause bacterial septicemia. Some effects of septicemia are: Very high fever, pronounced weakness, chills, a blood pressure drop, and local infections throughout the body as the bacteria spreads. If septicemia is not treated right away, it can lead to septic shock, which can be fatal (at least 50% of cases). The elderly are at a higher risk for developing septicemia, because they may have underlying diseases like diabetes, which make them more likely to get infections.

SHIGA TOXIN TESTS

Shiga toxin tests are used to isolate and confirm the presence of microorganisms that produce Shiga toxins. A fresh stool specimen should be collected in 3-tube stool kit as soon as possible after onset of diarrhea and prior to beginning antibiotic therapy. The specimen may be maintained at room temperature for 24 hours and under refrigeration for 2 days. The screening may be done through PCR, EIA, or culture. Shiga testing kits, such as BioStar® OIA SHIGATOX test, are available commercially to help identify strains. Identification of some strains of Shiga toxin–producing microorganisms may require sending the sample to a state public health laboratory. For example, some strains of *E. coli* are Shiga-producing, and stool cultures are not able to detect all strains, so EIAs, which are not always readily available because of cost, are required for testing.

NEISSERIACEAE

The family of bacteria *Neisseriaceae* is gram-negative cocci that are shaped like kidney beans and prosper at a temperature of 37°C in an environment with carbon dioxide levels between five and 10%. This bacteria is subject to rapid drying and will die at cold temperatures. *Neisseriaceae* are located in the bacterial flora of the respiratory and urogenital systems, as well as in the stomach. These bacteria are oxidase positive.

MEDIA UPON WHICH COCCI BACTERIA GROWS

1. *Staphylococcus aureus*: Will grow on a wide variety of media, including mannitol salt agar
2. *Streptococcus pneumoniae*: 5% sheep's blood agar with five to 10% carbon dioxide
3. *Neisseria gonorrhoeae*: Chocolate, Martin-Lewis, New York City, GC-Lect, and Thayer-Martin agar
4. Neisseria meningitides: Blood agar
5. Moraxella catarrhalis: Nutrients agars

DISEASES OR CONDITIONS ASSOCIATED WITH SHIGELLA, KLEBSIELLA, SALMONELLA TYPHI, PSEUDOMONAS AERUGINOSA, AND STENOTROPHOMONAS MALTOPHILIA

1. *Shigella*: Bacterial dysentery, otherwise known as shigellosis
2. *Klebsiella*: Pneumonia and urinary tract infections
3. Salmonella typhi: Typhoid fever
4. *Pseudomonas aeruginosa*: Swimmer's ear, ear infections, respiratory tract infections, burn wound infections, and eye infections
5. *Stenotrophomonas maltophilia*: Urinary tract infections, pneumonia, and wound infections

Specimen Needed for Laboratory Analysis When Testing for *Group A Streptococcus*, *Klebsiella Pneumoniae*, *Salmonella spp.*, *Gardnerella Vaginalis*, *Legionella Pneumophilia*, and *Neisseria Gonorrhoeae*

1. Group A *Streptococcus*: Throat culture
2. Klebsiella pneumoniae: Sputum specimen
3. Salmonella spp.: Stool sample
4. *Gardnerella vaginalis*: Specimen from genital tract
5. Legionella pneumophilia: Sputum specimen
6. *Neisseria gonorrhoeae*: Specimen from genital tract

GROUPING MYCOBACTERIA

There are a few different ways to classify the members of the genus *Mycobacterium*. For one, they may be classified according to photo reactivity. By this standard, there are three classes: photochromogens, which produce orange and yellow pigments when exposed to light;

scotochromogens, which produce yellow and orange pigments in both light and dark; and nonchromogens, which do not produce any pigments in either light or dark. These bacteria may also be classified according to morphology, given that each individual member has a distinctive colony appearance. Finally, mycobacteria may be classified according to their rate of growth.

USING TRIPLE SUGAR IRON AGAR (TSI) TEST IN ENTERIC IDENTIFICATION

Laboratory technicians often use the triple sugar iron agar test to differentiate among various kinds of *Enterobacteriaceae* bacteria. This is an especially useful test, because it can give data on glucose fermentation, lactose fermentation, sucrose fermentation and H_2S formation. There are four possible results for a TSI test:

- yellow (acid) deep: yellow bacteria, glucose positive
- yellow slant (acid): light yellow bacteria, sucrose or lactose positive
- alkaline slant/alkaline deep: bacteria are not members of *Enterobacteriaceae*, since they are not fermenters
- alkaline slant/acid deep: red or yellow bacteria, glucose positive and non-lactose fermenters

HOW VARIOUS ANTIBIOTICS WORK

1. Macrolides: Interferes with the protein synthesis of bacteria
2. Glycopeptides: Obstructs the formation of bacterial cell walls, by preventing the synthesis of peptidoglycans
3. Quinolones: Limits the activity of bacterial DNA
4. Sulfonamides: Obstructs the synthesis of bacteria
5. Aminoglycosides:O obstructs protein synthesis in both gram-positive and gram-negative bacteria
6. Beta-lactam antibiotics: Prevent the synthesis of bacterial cell walls

FECAL OCCULT BLOOD AND IMMUNOCHEMICAL TESTS

Stool may be examined macroscopically for volume, odor, color, consistency, mucus, and microscopically to identify the presence of cells (leukocytes, epithelial cells) and other materials (meat fibers). **Tests for occult blood** commonly include:

- **Fecal occult blood test (FOBT):** This test detects blood that has occurred from anywhere in the digestive tract because the blood reacts to the guaiac the test card is coated with. This test cannot distinguish between bleeding from the upper GI tract and the lower GI tract, so it is less specific than the FIT.
- **Fecal immunochemical test (FIT):** This test detects blood in the stool from lower GI bleeding through the use of antibodies against human hemoglobin (so it does not react to animal hemoglobin from ingested meats). FIT does not detect upper GI bleeding because the hemoglobin has been broken down by the digestive process by the time it reaches the rectum and is expelled.

MRSA AND ITS IMPORTANCE IN HEALTHCARE-ASSOCIATED INFECTIONS (HAIS)

Methicillin-resistant *Staphylococcus aureus* (MRSA) was first identified in 1961 in Europe after the development and overuse of synthetic penicillins caused *Staphylococcus aureus* to mutate into resistant strains. Since 1961, MRSA has infected millions of people worldwide. MRSA is resistant to methicillin and other β-lactam antibiotics, such as amoxicillin and oxacillin, and sometimes other classes of antibiotics. *Staphylococcus* is able to form biofilms, which aids in resistance. Healthcare-associated MRSA infections most commonly involve surgical sites, urinary tract, blood stream, and lungs (pneumonia). Because of increased awareness and better practices, MRSA HAIs decreased by 54% between 2004 and 2011 but still pose a threat to patients because of the severity of some infections and the risk of resistance to other drugs. Community-acquired MRSA most commonly results in skin infections, such as folliculitis, and can easily spread to others where groups of people are in close contact, such as in day cares, gyms, schools, and barracks.

MULTI-DRUG-RESISTANT ORGANISMS

Multi-drug-resistant organisms (MDRO): MDROs are those that have mutated and developed forms that are resistant to multiple antibiotics. Initially, resistance developed to one class of antibiotics, such as β-lactams, which resulted in methicillin-resistant *Staphylococcus aureus* infections and penicillin-resistant *Streptococcus pneumoniae*, but bacteria continued to mutate, becoming resistant to more classes of antibiotics and severely limiting the antibiotic arsenal needed for treatment. Of current concern is extended-spectrum beta-lactamases (ESBLs), resistant to cephalosporins and monobactams; and multi-drug-resistant tuberculosis (MDR).

VANCOMYCIN-RESISTANT *ENTEROCOCCUS*

Vancomycin-resistant *Enterococcus* (VRE): Up until the 1980s, most enterococci responded to vancomycin, a strong antibiotic, but the increased use of antibiotics for all types of infection resulted in mutations that rendered some enterococci species vancomycin-resistant (VRE), leaving few options for treatment of severe infection. There are currently 6 different forms (A-G) of vancomycin resistance. For example, the Van-A form is resistant to vancomycin and teicoplanin (an alternative antibiotic for severe infections).

TYPES, CLASSIFICATIONS, DESCRIPTION, AND IDENTIFICATION OF PARASITES IN CLINICAL SPECIMENS

PARASITES: PROTISTS (PROTOZOA—ONE-CELLED ANIMAL FORM)

Intestinal flagellates: Giardia lamblia, Trichomonas vaginalis, Dientamoeba fragilis.	Contain one or more flagella (whip-like tails), and some have undulating membrane.	Identify cysts or trophozoites in fecal smears, PCR, EIA, antigen detection.
Hemoflagellates: Trypanosoma, Leishmania, Trypanosoma cruzi		
Intestinal amoebas: Entamoeba histolytica, Balantidium coli	Have 3 stages: amoeba, inactive cyst, and intermediate precyst. Move with pseudopodia.	Identify cysts in stool specimen, EIA, antigen detection, PCR.
Blood apicomplexa/sporozoa: Plasmodium vivax, ovale, malariae, and falciparum; Isospora belli; Babesia microti, sarcocystis spp.; Cryptosporidium spp; Toxoplasma gondii	Spore-forming with organelle to penetrate host cell.	Plasmodium: Thick and thin Giemsa-stained blood film to identify organisms, antigen-capture tests. Others: Identify oocysts in fresh stool, PCR, EIA, DFA, GPP.
Microsporida: Encephalitozoon hellum, Enterocytozoon bieneusi, encephalitozoon intestinalis	One-celled spore with tubular polar filament to inject sporoplasm into host where it develops.	Electron microscopy to identify spore, nuclei, and polar filament.

Ciliates: Balantidium coli	Organism with cilia in rows/patches and 2 kinds of nuclei.	Identifying cysts or trophozoites in stool.

HELMINTHS (PARASITIC WORMS)

Nematoda (Round worms): *Ascaris lumbricoides, Anisakis* spp. (cod/herring worms), *Enterobius vermicularis* (pinworms), *Strongyloides stercoralis, Ancylostoma duodenale/Necator americanus* (hookworm)	Size varies from 0.3 mm to 8 m, long, narrow non-segmented cylindrical body. Stages include egg, larva filariform and/or rhabditiform, and adult.	Identify eggs, parasites, or larvae in stool specimen.
		Pinworms: Cellophane tape test.
Cestoda (Tapeworms) *Hymenolepis nana* (dwarf tapeworm), *Taenia saginata* (beef tapeworm, *Taenia solium* (pork tapeworm), *Diphyllobothrium latum* (fish tapeworm)	Long, flat, segmented worms with scolex (head/sucker), neck, and strobila (segments).	Identify proglottids and eggs or scolex in stool specimen.
	Stages include egg/gravid proglottids, oncosphere, cysticercus, cysticercoid, and adult.	
Trematoda (flatworms/flukes): *Fasciolopsis buski, Heterophyes, Schistosoma* spp.	Flat, leaf-shaped, non-segmented worms. Stages may include egg, miracidium, sporocyst, redia, cercariae, metacercariae, excyst, and adult.	Identify eggs in stool specimen.

STRING TEST

The string test, sometimes referred to as the Entero-test, is used to help determine the presence of a parasitic infection. Usually, stool samples are examined first for parasites. If no parasites are found and the patient is still symptomatic, the string test is employed. Attach a string to a weighted gelatin capsule and observe the patient as he/she swallows it. Approximately four hours later, retrieve the string through the patient's mouth. Examine any mucus from the intestines that is attached to the string under a microscope. Any parasites and/or eggs that are present can then be seen. This test is not very common, but it can help determine the presence of various parasites, such as *Giardia lamblia*, a common cause of gastrointestinal disease.

ENTEROBIASIS TAPE TEST

The enterobiasis tape test is used to discover pinworms (enterobiasis). Use a flashlight and sticky tape to gather pinworms and pinworm eggs from the patient's anus as he/she sleeps. If the patient wishes to do it, it must be done first thing in the morning because pinworms tend to deposit eggs near the anus overnight, and disappear back into the rectum. Touch the sticky side of the tape onto a clean glass slide, and examine it under the microscope. Any pinworms or pinworm eggs that are present will be seen at low magnification. Sometimes, more than one enterobiasis tape test needs to be done to achieve accurate results. Performing the test for three days straight is sufficient. If pinworms or their eggs are found, the infection is usually treated with the Mebendazole.

CONTROLLING INFECTION OF VARIOUS PARASITES

1. Infection with *Toxoplasma gondii* (Toxoplasmosis) can best be prevented by either cooking all meat products thoroughly or by washing one's hands after touching cat feces or cleaning cat litter boxes.

2. Infection with *Necator americanus*, a hookworm, can best be prevented by disposing of human waste (feces) in a sanitary manner.
3. Infection with *Enterobius vermicularis*, a pinworm, can best be prevented by following good personal hygiene practices. Washing one's hands before eating meals or after using the bathroom can help prevent infection by this parasite.
4. Infection with *Trichinella spiralis* (Trichinosis) can best be prevented by cooking all pork and wild game products thoroughly. This cooking will destroy any parasite encysted in the pork muscle or wild game.

HELMINTHS

Helminths are parasitic worms that live in humans, primarily in the intestines. There are a variety of helminths, including roundworms, tapeworms, pinworms, flukes, and the worm *Trichinella spiralis*, which is responsible for causing trichinosis. Eggs from helminthes can contaminate a variety of things, including feces, pets and other animals, water, air, food, and surfaces like toilet seats. Eggs of helminths usually enter a human via the anus, the nose, or the mouth, and they then travel to the intestines, where they hatch, grow, and multiply. The presence of helminths can be determined in most cases by examining stool samples of suspected infected individuals. Drugs known as vermifuges can be used to treat infections from helminth worms. To prevent infection from helminths, thoroughly cook meats, keep a clean kitchen and bathroom, and wash hands frequently.

ETIOLOGIC AGENTS OF VARIOUS DISEASES

Disease	Etiologic Agents
sleeping sickness	*Trypanosoma rhodesiense* or *Trypanosoma gambiense*
malaria	*Plasmodium sp.*, including *P. falciparum*, *P. ovale*, *P. vivax*, and *P. malariae*, among others
elephantiasis	a roundworm, either *Wuchereria bancrofti* or *Brugia malayi*
Katayama fever (schistosomiasis)	a blood fluke, namely *Schistosoma mansoni*, *Schistosoma haematobium*, or *Schistosoma japonicum*
scabies	a mite, *Sarcoptes scabiei*
isosporiasis	*Isosporiasis belli*
toxoplasmosis	*Toxoplasma gondii*

VECTORS FOR CHAGAS' DISEASE, *PLASMODIUM VIVAX*, *LOA LOA*, *BABESIA SP.*, AND TRICHINOSIS

1. The most important vector for Chagas' disease is a reduviid bug, also known as a kissing bug. The most common reduviid bugs implicated in Chagas' disease are *Rhodnius prolixus* and *Triatoma infestans*. A reduviid bug infected with the parasite, Trypanosoma *cruzi* deposits fecal material on the skin of a person while he/she is sleeping. The person then rubs the fecal matter into their mouth, nose, eyes, or an open wound.
2. The most important vector for *Plasmodium vivax* is an infected mosquito. Most often, the mosquito is a female Anopheles mosquito. The mosquito infected with *Plasmodium vivax* bites a human, thereby transmitting the parasite to the human. *Plasmodium vivax* is the number one cause of malaria in humans.

Copyright © Mometrix Media. You have been licensed one copy of this document for personal use only. Any other reproduction or redistribution is strictly prohibited. All rights reserved.

3. The most important vector for *loa loa* are horsefly, mango fly (genus Chrysops) and deer fly. Loa loa is a filarial worm, and when an infected horsefly or deerfly bites a human, the parasitic worm can then be transmitted to the human.
4. The most important vector of Babesia sp. is a deer tick, namely *Ixodes dammini* that bites a human, thereby transmitting the parasite to the human's bloodstream. Here the parasite multiplies, and the disease that is caused due to such a bite is babesiosis.
5. The most important vector for trichinosis is undercooked pork or wild game infected with the larvae of a round worm, *Trichinella spiralis*. If the pork or wild game were thoroughly cooked, the transmission of the parasite to humans would be greatly reduced.

TYPE(S) ASSOCIATED WITH VARIOUS PARASITES

1. Trichomonas: Vaginal, mouth, nasal, urethral, urine
2. Acanthamoeba: Tissue samples, eye scrapings
3. Onchocerca: Skin samples, blood samples
4. Entamoeba: Nasal samples, mouth samples, sputum samples
5. Naegleria: Nasal samples, tissue samples, mouth samples

DIAGNOSTIC TESTS USED IN THE IDENTIFICATION OF PARASITES

1. Direct agglutination test (DAT): Used to diagnose leishmaniasis and Chagas' disease
2. Direct fluorescent antibody (DFA) test: Used to identify *Trichomonas vaginalis*
3. Gel diffusion precipitin (GDP) test: Used to diagnose and identify amoebic infections
4. Indirect immunofluorescent antibody (IFA) test: Used to diagnose malaria, amoebic infection, toxoplasmosis, and schistosome infections
5. Complement fixation (CF): Used to diagnose pneumocystosis, Chagas' disease, and leishmaniasis

MORPHOLOGY OF FILARIAE

1. *Brugia malayi*: a filarial nematode ranging from 200 to 300 μm long, with a sheath and two nuclei in its tail; can result in Malayan filiaris and elephantiasis, when there are lesions in the lymphatic system
2. *Loa Loa*: a filarial nematode between 250 and 300 μm long, with a sheath and two nuclei in its tail; transmitted by deer fly bite, this nematode is responsible for infections in the subcutaneous tissue and in the conjunctival lining of the eye
3. *Onchocerca volvulus*: a filarial nematode ranging from 150 to 360 μm long, with a sheath but no nuclei in its tail; transmitted by the blackfly, this nematode is responsible for severe eye infections, often resulting in blindness

MYCOLOGICAL ORGANISMS (FUNGI)

Most fungi are aerobic and have at least 1 nucleus. Fungi secrete enzymes and are part of natural microbial flora. Yeasts: Single cell spherical/ellipsoid 3-15 μm in diameter. Some produce buds and chains of buds called pseudohyphae. Colonies are 1-3 mm in size, cream colored. Molds: Growth is per multicellular filamentous colonies with branching intertwined tubules called hyphae, which are 2-10 μm in diameter. Fungi may be classified in a number of ways, but for medical purposes classification according to the site of infection is most common. Fungi are often described by appearance as cottony, powdery, velvety, or glabrous (waxy).

Superficial mycoses	Pityriasis versicolor (*Malassezia* spp, tinea nigra, piedra)	Invade superficial layers of skin and hair shaft.

Cutaneous mycoses	Tinea corporis, tinea pedis, tinea cruris, tinea capitis, tinea barbae, tinea unguium, dermatophytid	Infect superficial keratinized tissue, such as hair, skin, and nails. Unable to grow if serum is present or temperature is ≥37°C.
Subcutaneous mycoses	*Sporothrix schenckii*, chromoblastomycosis, phaeohyphomycosis, mycetoma, *Coccidioides immitis, Coccidioides posadasii*	Normally grow in soil or vegetation and infect through traumatic inoculation. Infections are usually subcutaneous but in rare cases spread systemically.
Endemic mycoses	Coccidioidomycosis, histoplasmosis, blastomycosis, paracoccidioidomycosis, candidiasis, aspergillosis, sporotrichosis	Most infections result from inhalation in immunocompromised individuals. Infections cause inflammatory response and production of cell-mediated immunity and antibodies.

MYCOLOGICAL PROCEDURES TO IDENTIFY FUNGI

Exoantigen test	The exoantigen test is a gel immunodiffusion precipitin test in which soluble antigens produced by fungi grown in broth media react with anti-serum (produced from rabbits injected with antigens), allowing for identification of dimorphic fungi. Fungi are identified according the presence of specific antigens. This test has been generally supplanted by DNA probe testing.
DNA probe	DNA probe testing is more efficient and less time-consuming than the exoantigen test and poses les risk to laboratory workers. A DNA probe is a DNA fragment that is labeled with a fluorescent or radioactive material and can recognize genes in DNA sequences of specific organisms. Procedures vary widely, depending upon the specific type of test, but PCR probe-based tests are available for mycological studies to identify pathogenic fungi.

KOH TEST

The KOH (potassium hydroxide) test is the first that should be used to identify fungi in a sample of human skin, nails, tissue, or hair. The KOH test dissolves the human cells, leaving only the fungal cells for examination. Scrape a sample of human cells suspected to contain a fungus onto a laboratory slide. Add several drops of 10% KOH in water to the slide. Cover the slide with a coverslip. Warm the slide in a Bunsen burner flame, but do not boil it. Examine it under a microscope. The KOH will have dissolved the human cells. Any visible cells are fungal. The differences in the composition of the cell walls of human and fungal cells allow for this reaction with the KOH solution.

DERMATOPHYTES

Dermatophytes are a type of pathogenic and parasitic fungi. These fungi most often cause infections of skin, hair, and nails, on humans and other animals. Two types of infections caused by dermatophytes are tinea and ringworm. There are three genera of dermatophytes: *Epidermophyton*, *Microsporum*, and *Trichophyton*. In the laboratory, they can be identified on Sabouraud's agar. Examination of the morphology of the macroconidia and the microconidia produced is a very reliable method for identification of dermatophytes. Sometimes, stimulating spore production in the sample can also be useful in dermatophyte identification. However, coloring and texture of the fungi can be variable, so these characteristics are not very reliable in dermatophyte identification.

KERATITIS

Keratitis is inflammation or lesion of the cornea, causing pain, problems with sight, blindness, or other eye damage. Keratitis can occur after injury to the eye, and can either be deep or superficial in nature. Superficial keratitis does not leave a scar on the cornea; however, deep keratitis does tend to leave a scar on the cornea, and this can have a permanent effect on the patient's vision. Fungal keratitis is caused by the fungus *Fusarium*, which is prevalent in plants and soils. It also is a plant pathogen, in addition to the effects it has on human health. The doctor will provide you with corneal scrapings to determine the presence of *Fusarium* in a case of suspected fungal keratitis. Stain the sample and culture it on Sabouraud's agar.

TYPES OF FUNGAL MEDIA

1. Brain heart infusion agar with blood (BHIB): grows most varieties of fungi, especially on sterile human body sites; composed of brain heart infusion and sheep's blood
2. Sabouraud brain heart infusion agar (SABHI): grows most varieties of fungi, and will also grow bacteria
3. Dermatophyte test medium (DTM): good for growing dermatophytes, or skin fungi; antibiotics within the substance obstruct bacterial growth and aid in the development of specific fungi
4. Cornmeal tween 80: a differential agar used to distinguish varieties of *Candida*
5. Birdseed agar: a differential agar used to grow *Cryptococcus neoformans*
6. Potato dextrose agar: a differential agar used to enhance pigmentation of the fungus *Trichophyton rubrum*
7. Cottonseed agar: differential agar used to speed the transition from mold to yeast in the fungi *Blastomyces dermatitidis*

TRICHOPHYTON

The genus of fungi known as *Trichophyton* has both macroconidia and microconidia. The macroconidia are few in number and resemble pencils with thin, smooth walls. The microconidia, meanwhile, are clustered together like grapes and are either round or oblong. All the members of this genus of fungi show up well on a Sabouraud brain heart infusion agar (SABHI), typically between seven and 10 days after initiation. The fungi will either appear as white and fluffy colonies or as granular red or beige colonies with a red, brown, or yellow reverse color.

COLONY OF ASPERGILLUS

The fungi *Aspergillus* will grow within 48 hours on a SABHI culture, with the colonies being granular, fluffy, or powdery, and of various colors. *Aspergillus flavus* colonies are brown and green, with a brownish red reverse color; *Aspergillus terreus* colonies are yellow or green, with a yellow reverse color; *Aspergillus fumigatus* colonies are gray or green, with a beige reverse color; and *Aspergillus niger* colonies are yellow or black, with a yellow reverse color. This fungus is responsible for aspergillosis, which can damage the respiratory system, skin, heart, and central nervous system.

IDENTIFICATION OF FUNGI

1. Wright stain: used to distinguish the yeast forms of the blood fungus *Histoplasma capsulatum*
2. Gram stain: used to distinguish *Cryptococcus neoformans*

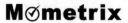

3. India ink: used to distinguish the capsules around Cryptococcus neoformans in cerebral spinal fluid
4. Calcofluor white stain: used to delineate the cell walls of a fungus

WESTERN BLOT TEST

The Western blot test is used in the laboratory to help confirm or deny the presence of HIV virus. Unlike the Southern blot and Northern blot tests, this test can test for both DNA and RNA protein fragments. Gel electrophoresis is used to separate these fragments of the viruses' DNA and RNA, and then they are covered with a membrane composed of nitrocellulose. The patient's serum is reacted with these separated DNA and RNA fragments. If the patient's serum contains antibodies for the HIV virus, those antibodies will bind to the DNA and RNA fragments present. This binding will produce a characteristic pattern (referred to as the characteristic blot), which can then be visualized. This pattern can then confirm the presence of the HIV virus in the patient's blood serum.

SOUTHERN BLOT TEST

The Southern blot test is used to identify DNA (deoxyribonucleic acid) fragments in the laboratory. In this test, gel electrophoresis is used to separate fragments of DNA. Then, these fragments are covered with a membrane consisting of nitrocellulose. Finally, a specific probe is used to identify the fragments of DNA.

NORTHERN BLOT TEST

The Northern blot test is used to identify RNA (ribonucleic acid) sequences in the laboratory. First, fragments of RNA are separated using gel electrophoresis. Then, as in the Southern blot test, the fragments are covered with a nitrocellulose membrane. Lastly, a specific probe for this procedure is used to identify the RNA sequences present.

IDENTIFYING THE PRESENCE OF RICKETTSIA USING GIMENEZ STAIN

The Gimenez stain is a stain that can be used to identify the presence of Rickettsia in a sample. Apply carbol-fuchsin solution to an air-dried smear for approximately one to two minutes. Wash the smear with tap water. Apply a malachite green solution to the smear for approximately six to nine seconds. Finally, wash the smear once again with tap water. Observe the smear under the microscope. The carbol-fuchsin solution will have colored the Rickettsia that are present a red, pink, or magenta color. The counterstain, the malachite green solution, will have colored the background of the sample a bluish-green color. The Rickettsia often will be rod shaped.

RICKETTSIA

Rickettsia is a genus of bacteria. These bacteria are carried by fleas, ticks, and lice and transmitted to humans. Members of the genus Rickettsia are gram-negative, non-motile, and they do not form spores. They can have a variety of bacteria shapes, ranging from thread-like to cocci to rods. They are also very small in size, and they need a living host to grow and multiply. Therefore, in the laboratory, they have to be grown in living embryo or tissue cultures. Chicken embryos can be used for this purpose. Some diseases that are caused by members of the genus Rickettsia include typhus, scrub typhus, and spotted fever. They can also cause a variety of diseases in plants as well. In humans, diseases caused by Rickettsia often respond well to tetracycline antibiotics.

RHINOVIRUS

Rhinoviruses are a particular genus of the family of viruses, Picornaviridae. There are at least 113 different types of rhinoviruses that affect humans. Rhinoviruses contain ribonucleic acid (RNA), and they are very small in size, on the order of 17 to 30 nanometers. Rhinoviruses are responsible for causing many disorders of the respiratory system, including the common cold. Rhinoviruses are transmitted to the human respiratory tract via breathing in airborne droplets, or by touching one's eyes, mouth, or nose with fingers or hands that have been exposed to airborne droplets containing the rhinovirus. Different rhinoviruses are prevalent during different times of the year in a particular location, but more than one type of rhinovirus can be prevalent at a given time. Because of the many different types of rhinoviruses, finding a vaccine has been difficult, and none exists at this time. Rhinoviruses affect more humans than all other viruses, making them the most common type of virus.

CAUSATIVE AGENTS OF VARIOUS DISEASES

Disease	Causative Agents
scrub typhus	*Rickettsia tsutsugamushi*
Rocky Mountain spotted fever	*Rickettsia rickettsia*
rickettsial pox	*Rickettsia akari*
murine typhus	*Rickettsia typhi*
Oroya fever	*Bartonella bacilliformis*
molluscum contagiosum	poxvirus
conjunctivitis	adenovirus
yellow fever	arbovirus
human hand, foot, and mouth disease	Coxsackie virus
hepatitis A	Picorna virus
AIDS	human immunodeficiency virus

KOPLIK'S SPOTS, NEGRI BODIES, AND DANE PARTICLE

1. Koplik's spots are characteristic of the measles (rubeola). They are small red spots or lesions that contain a bluish-white colored speck at their center. They are found in the mouth of an infected person. Because they do not last for a long time, they may not even be noted.
2. Negri bodies are characteristic of rabies. They are inclusions in the cytoplasm of nerve cells (neurons) that have been infected with the rabies virus. They are acidophilic (stain well with acid dyes), and they have a diameter of approximately 2—10 μm.
3. The Dane particle is the causative agent of type B hepatitis. The inner Dane particle contains DNA, and the outer layer of the particle contains the surface antigen for the hepatitis B virus. Dane particles are approximately 42 nm in diameter.

MEASLES

The measles is a virus that most often affects children of school age, and most often children in developing countries. In the United States, vaccination against the measles in early childhood is recommended. The measles is easily spread from human to human, and it enters the body through the respiratory system by inhalation. The virus multiplies in the respiratory system, and spreads through the circulatory system. Some of the symptoms of the measles are: A characteristic body rash that appears within 14 days of being infected, a high fever, red eyes, sneezing, and cough. Also, Koplik's spots may be seen. These spots are small and reddish with a bluish-white spot in their centers, and appear in the mouth, but since they only persist for a short time, their presence may not be noted. Complications, such as pneumonia, can arise from the measles. The presence of measles IgM antibodies can be detected through serum analysis. Most cases of the measles last about seven to ten days.

TYPES OF SAMPLES TO TEST FOR GASTROENTERITIS, ENCEPHALITIS, VIRAL MENINGITIS, AND CUTANEOUS RASHES

1. Gastroenteritis: stool samples and/or rectal swabs; may be caused by adenovirus or calicivirus
2. Encephalitis: brain biopsy or serum sample; may be caused by herpes simplex virus one (HSV-1), arbovirus, or varicella-zoster virus (VZV)
3. Viral meningitis: urine samples, serum samples, stool samples, throat swabs, or cerebral spinal fluid samples; may be caused by VZV, herpes simplex virus two (HSV-2), enterovirus, mumps, or lymphocytic choriomeningitis virus
4. Cutaneous rashes: throat swabs, urine samples, stool samples, or serum samples; may be caused by HSV-1, HSV-2, measles, rubella, Epstein-Barr virus, parvovirus B-19, enterovirus, echovirus, and cytomegalovirus

CHICKENPOX VS. SHINGLES

Both chickenpox and shingles are caused by the varicella-zoster virus, which is a kind of herpesvirus 90 to 100 nanometers large. These viruses are icosahedral in shape and contain DNA. Shingles mainly occurs in adult humans and is considered to be a reactivation of the chickenpox virus that takes place in the peripheral or cranial nerves. Symptoms include pain and skin vesicles, which, if left untreated, can deteriorate into eye problems and central nervous system disorders. Chickenpox typically affects children, and has a characteristic rash as its main symptom. Chickenpox is usually spread by means of airborne droplets.

Size and Shape of Orthomyxovirus, Paramyxovirus, Retrovirus, Rhabdovirus, Reovirus, and Herpesvirus

1. Orthomyxovirus: 75 to 125 nm; contain RNA; helix-shaped; one example is influenza
2. Paramyxovirus: 150 to 300 nm; contain RNA; helix-shaped; one common example is mumps
3. Retrovirus: 80 to 130 nm; contain RNA; icosahedral in shape; one common example is HIV
4. Rhabdovirus: 150 to 350 nm; bullet-shaped; contain RNA; one common example is rabies
5. Reovirus: 50 to 80 nm; contain RNA; icosahedral shape; one common example is rotavirus
6. Herpes virus: 90 to 100 nm; contain DNA; icosahedral shape; one common example is herpes simplex virus

HEPATITIS A VIRUS AND HEPATITIS B VIRUS

1. Hepatitis A virus (HAV): contains RNA, has icosahedral shape; 24 to 30 nm in size, with no envelope; causes nausea, jaundice, and anorexia; 15- to 40-day incubation period, with low mortality rate; transmitted fecal to oral, typically because of poor food sanitation practices
2. Hepatitis B virus (HBV): contains DNA, Dane particles, and an envelope; 42 to 47 nm; transmitted through contaminated body fluids, often during tattoos, needle sticks, and intravenous drug abuse; 50- to 80-day incubation period, occasionally leading to liver failure; vaccinations have been developed

Urinalysis and Body Fluids

ANURIA, OLIGURIA, POLYURIA, AND NOCTURIA

1. anuria: almost no urine discharge, usually due to renal failure or other kidney damage
2. oliguria: sharp decrease in urine discharge; typically caused by diarrhea, vomiting, perspiration, or other forms of dehydration
3. polyuria: sharp increase in urine discharge, to a level over 3 L per day; often caused by ingestion of diuretics, caffeine, alcohol, or by diabetes insipidus or mellitus
4. nocturia: nocturnal increase in urine discharge; often caused by a reduction in bladder capacity due to increased ingestion of fluids, pregnancy, or enlargement of the prostate gland

METHODS OF URINE COLLECTION

1. Glucose tolerance test: used to diagnose diabetes or to monitor a diabetic; urine collection every hour, for three hours
2. Void: also known as random sample; patient collects his or her own urine
3. Midstream clean catch: patient cleans pubic area and then collects sample in mid-urination
4. 24-hour: all urine output is collected over a 24-hour period
5. Suprapubic aspiration: a needle is placed into the bladder and urine is extracted
6. Two-hour postprandial: urine is collected two hours after a meal; often performed to measure levels of sugar

RENAL ANATOMY AND PHYSIOLOGY AND FORMATION OF URINE

The **kidneys** are located on the right and left sides posterior to the peritoneal cavity and are responsible for the fluid and acid-base balance in the body. The cortex (body) is encased in a capsule. Inside the cortex are pyramids, papilla, major and minor calyces, and renal pelvis leading to the ureter that carries urine to the bladder. The nephron is the functional unit responsible for filtering the blood (about 1200 mL/min) and removing waste products. The nephron includes:

-   Glomerulus (capillaries surrounded by Bowman's capsule): Fluids and solutes move from the blood across capillary membranes into Bowman's capsule but plasma proteins and blood cells stay in the blood because they are too large.
-   Bowman's capsule: Glomerular filtrate (similar to plasma) moves into proximal convoluted tubule.
-   Proximal convoluted tubule: Water and electrolytes reabsorbed.
-   Loop of Henle: Solutes, including glucose, reabsorbed.
-   Distal convoluted tubule: Sodium and water reabsorbed according to levels of antidiuretic hormone (ADH) (from pituitary gland) and aldosterone (from adrenal cortex).
-   Collecting duct: Carries urine into calyces of kidney for excretion.

PHYSICAL AND CHEMICAL PROPERTIES OF URINE

Color	Pale yellow/ amber and darkens when urine is concentrated or other substances (such as blood or bile) or present.
Appearance	Clear but may be slightly cloudy.
Odor	Slight. Bacteria may give urine a foul smell, depending upon the organism. Some foods, such as asparagus, change odor.
Specific gravity	1.015 to 1.025. May increase if protein levels increase or if there is fever, vomiting, or dehydration.

pH	Usually ranges between 4.5 and 8, with average of 5 to 6.
Sediment	Red cell casts from acute infections, broad casts from kidney disorders, and white cell casts from pyelonephritis. Leukocytes >10/ml³ are present with urinary tract infections.
Glucose, ketones, protein, blood, bilirubin, and nitrate	Negative. Urine glucose may increase with infection (with normal blood glucose). Frank blood may be caused by some parasites and diseases but also by drugs, smoking, excessive exercise, and menstrual fluids. Increased red blood cells may result from lower urinary tract infections.
Urobilinogen	0.1-1.0 units. Increased in liver disease.

BENEDICT'S TEST

Benedict's test is a laboratory test that is used to determine the presence of reducing substances in a urine sample. Some reducing substances that can be present in urine include glucose (which can be indicative of diabetes), other reducing sugars such as lactose and galactose, creatinine, uric acid, or ascorbic acid. The test can tell a technician or a doctor if reducing substances are present in the urine sample, but the test itself is nonspecific. In other words, the test cannot determine the specific reducing substance present. To perform the test, Benedict's reagent (a solution of copper sulfate, sodium carbonate, and sodium citrate) is added to a urine sample, and the mixture is heated. A red, yellow, or orange precipitate is indicative of the presence of a reducing substance in the urine. The precipitate is formed because the copper sulfate in the Benedict's reagent is reduced by any reducing substance contained in the urine.

ADDIS COUNT PROCEDURE

The Addis count is a laboratory technique to calculate the number of formed elements in a urine sample. The formed elements include blood cells (white blood cells and red blood cells) and casts. In this test, a twelve hour urine specimen is collected. Formalin is used as a preservative for the urine sample. After the twelve hour period, a specified quantity of the urine specimen is put in a centrifuge. Part of any resuspended urine sediment is then placed into a Neubauer blood-counting chamber. The squares of the blood-counting chamber are then examined. Any formed elements, such as casts, white blood cells, or red blood cells, that are present are counted. The total number of formed elements in the entire urine sample is then calculated. This test can be used on the urine of patients that have kidney disease.

URINALYSIS PROCEDURES

pH	Insert indicator paper or reagent strip into urine, remove excess, wait time according to manufacturer's guidelines, and compare to color chart.
Glucose	Use reagent strip OR place 5 mL of Benedict solution in test tube and 8 drops of urine, and mix. Boil solution for 2 minutes with Bunsen burner or spirit lamp with tube at about 45° angle or place tube in boiling water for 5 minutes. Cool tube and check color for amount of glucose with blue equal to 1+ and orange/red, 4+.
Nitrate/ Nitrite	Enzymes produced by bacteria change nitrate into nitrite, which is measured as an indirect method to detect UTI. Urine must have been in bladder for at least 4 hours, so first morning sample is usually used. Dip reagent strip in the urine sample and read results at 30 to 60 seconds and match against color chart with positive findings indicated by change to light to dark pink.

Bilirubin	Protect urine specimen from light and examine when fresh. Dip reagent strip in urine and read test results at 30 to 60 seconds and match against color chart with colors ranging from buff (1+) to tan/purple (3+) for positive reaction OR use Ictotest®.
Urobilinogen	Test fresh specimen between 2 and 4 PM (peak levels), especially for liver function testing. Dip reagent strip in the urine sample, read results at 30 to 60 seconds, and match to color chart with positive color changes ranging from peach-colored (0.2 mg/dL) to bright pink (8 mg/dL).
Protein	Use reagent strip OR place 5 mL of urine in a test tube and add 2 drops of sulfosalicylic acid. Observe for formation of white precipitate and as negative or from + to ++++ (trace to large amount) depending on the amount of precipitate.
Ketones	Use Acetest® tablets OR dip ketone stick in urine, wait 15 seconds, and monitor color changes. Positive changes are light lavender (5 mg/dL) to purple (160 mg/dL).
Blood	Place 12 mL urine in conical tube, centrifuge 5 minutes (medium speed), pour off supernatant, shake tube, use pipette to remove 1 drop of sediment and place on slide for microscopic examination. RBCs appear colored (yellow/green).
Leukocyte esterase	Obtain clean catch urine sample in sterile container, dip reagent strip into urine and check color chart after 2 minutes. No color change is negative but shades of pink to purple indicate trace to large amounts.

HCG Hemagglutination Inhibition Test

The HCG hemagglutination test is used to determine pregnancy by examining a urine sample. Add a sample of urine to two drops of HCG antiserum. To this, add red blood cells that have been coated in HCG. If HCG is present in the urine sample, the HCG antiserum binds to the HCG present, therefore making it impossible for the HCG antiserum to react with the red blood cells coated in HCG. This leads to the red cells not agglutinating, and a donut shape consisting of red blood cells will form. This donut shape indicates HCG in the urine sample. However, if there is no HCG present in the urine sample, the HCG antiserum will bind with the HCG coated red blood cells. No donut pattern of red blood cells will form. Instead, there will be a diffuse pattern of red blood cells. This diffuse pattern indicates that no HCG is present in the urine sample. The patient is not pregnant, or is pregnant more than six months.

Confirmatory Urine Tests

Clinitest®	Confirms the presence of glucose in the urine. Drop alkaline copper reagent tables in a tube containing 5 drops of urine and 10 drops of distilled water, which will boil. Wait 15 seconds after boiling stops, gently shake tube, and check color against chart. Blue is negative and colors from green to orange indicate the presence of 1/4% (+) to 2% (++++) glucose.
Ictotest®	Confirms the presence of bilirubin in the urine. Place 10 drops of urine on a special absorbant mat, place a reagent table in the middle of the moistened are and then one drop of distilled water on the tablet. After 5 seconds, place another drop of distilled water on the table. Wait 60 seconds and observe the color about and under the tablet. Blue or purple color indicates the presence of bilirubin.

Acetest® (Acetone test)	Confirms the presence of ketones in the urine. Place tablet on clean dry white paper and place 1 drop of urine on top of tablet. Wait 30 seconds and check color against color chart. No change in color is negative and shades of lavender (light, medium, and dark) indicate small, moderate, and large amounts of ketones.
Sulfosalicylic acid (SSA)	Confirms the presence of protein in the urine. If urine is cloudy, centrifuge before test. Fill tube (10 × 75 mm) one-third full of urine and add one-third tube of 3% SSA solution. Cover with paraffin film/cap and mix by inverting. Check results by holding in front of lined/text test strip. If the lines/text are clear, the result is negative, slightly cloudy but lines/text visible, 1+; lines are visible but unable to read text, 2+; no lines/text visible, 3+; totally opaque/gelled, 4+.

EXAMPLE SITUATIONS AND POSSIBLE CAUSES

KETONE BODIES PRESENT IN URINE

The presence of ketone bodies in a urine or blood sample can be caused by diabetes mellitus or ketone producing diet. The ketone bodies are due to an excessive metabolism of fat because sugar cannot be utilized.

HUMAN CHORIONIC GONADOTROPIN PRESENT IN URINE

The presence of human chorionic gonadotropin (HCG) in the urine is due to pregnancy or testicular tumor. Within a week or two after conception, human chorionic gonadotropin is excreted into the urine, and it can be detected by a variety of laboratory techniques, including a radioimmunoassay.

URINE SEDIMENT THAT CONTAINS WHITE BLOOD CELLS

If white blood cells (usually neutrophils) are found in urine sediment that usually indicates the presence of a urinary tract or renal infection.

URINE THAT WHEN SHAKEN FORMS A YELLOW FOAM

Most samples of urine do not foam when shaken. However, if urine, when shaken, forms a yellow foam, that is due to an increased concentration of bilirubin in the urine.

ABNORMAL URINE COLORATIONS

1. Red: most commonly caused by blood; additional causes may be red blood cells, hemoglobin, myoglobin caused by muscle trauma
2. Dark yellow or amber: dehydration, infection, fever, or liver problems like hepatitis
3. Bright yellow or orange: caused by increased bilirubin, or by medications such as pyridium, which is used to treat urinary tract infections
4. Green: caused by presence of biliverdin, which is introduced by the breakdown of hemoglobin
5. Black or gray: presence of melanin or homogentisic acid resulting from a metabolic disorder

IMPORTANCE OF SPECIFIC GRAVITY IN URINALYSIS

Every urinalysis includes a measure of specific gravity, which indicates the degree to which the kidneys can reabsorb water and essential chemicals from the glomerular filtrate. Most kidney disorders impair this function immediately. Specific gravity tests also indicate whether hormone abnormalities or dehydration is present. A normal specific gravity will range from 1.001 to 1.035. If the specific gravity is greater than 1.010, it is called hypersthenuric urine. If the specific gravity is less than 1.010, it is called hyposthenuric urine. If the specific gravity is exactly 1.010, it is called isosthenuric urine.

REAGENT STRIPS

Lab technicians use reagent strips to examine the chemical composition of a urine sample. The following chemicals can be assessed: bilirubin, glucose, nitrite, blood, protein, white blood cells, ketones, and urobilinogen. Also, reagent strips can determine the specific gravity and pH of urine. These strips work as follows: they are dipped into the urine sample and change colors depending on the composition of the urine. As long as basic restrictions regarding room temperature and procedure are followed, these reagent strips are highly accurate.

URINE pH

Lab technicians often use pH reagent strips to determine the pH of a urine sample. Such a strip will contain bromethol blue and methyl red, and these chemicals will cause the strip to change colors depending on the pH of the urine. If the pH is 5.0, the strip will turn orange. As the pH of the urine increases, the resulting color on the strip will go from orange to yellow to green to blue. At a pH of 9.0, the strip will turn blue. Individuals will typically not have a pH lower than 6.0 except for first thing in the morning, or if they eat a high protein diet or have diabetes mellitus. Typical pH level will not be higher than 7.0 except in cases of renal tubular acidosis, urinary tract infection, or metabolic or respiratory alkalosis.

URINE COMPONENTS ASSOCIATED WITH REAGENT STRIPS

1. Sodium nitroprusside or nitro ferricyanide: Used to test for the presence of ketones in a sample of urine
2. Diazonium salt reaction: Used to test for the presence of bilirubin in a sample of urine
3. Tetrabromophenol blue: Used to test for the presence of abnormal levels of proteins in a sample of urine
4. Indoxyl carbonic acid ester: Used to test for the presence of white blood cells in a sample of urine

TERMS

Myoglobinuria: Condition in which urine contains myoglobin; often the result of muscle trauma, coma, or muscle destruction

Hematuria: Condition in which urine contains intact red blood cells; often caused by renal tumors, menstruation, or pregnancy

Hemoglobinuria: Condition in which urine contains hemoglobin; often caused by infections, transfusion reactions, hemolytic anemia, or burns

Ketonuria: Condition in which urine contains ketones; often the result of diabetes mellitus, dehydration, or chronic imbalance electrolytes

Bilirubinuria: Condition in which urine contains bilirubin; often caused by liver disease, hepatitis, or cirrhosis of the liver

URINE CASTS AND THEIR APPEARANCE UNDER A MICROSCOPE

1. White blood cell casts: Any cast containing white blood cells; indicates infection or inflammation
2. Red blood cell casts: Any casts that contain red blood cells, which will appear brown or yellow under a microscope; indicative of renal disease

3. Hyaline casts: The most common kind of cast, typically the result of renal disease, heart failure, or glomerulonephritis; often seen after stress, excessive exercise, or dehydration

URINE CRYSTALS AND THEIR APPEARANCE UNDER A MICROSCOPE

1. Cystine: Colorless, hexagonal plates
2. Tyrosine: Yellow or colorless thin needles
3. Cholesterol: Clear, flat rectangular crystals
4. Uric acid: Various; colorless or yellow, and shaped as cubes, diamonds, plates, or needles
5. Bilirubin: Yellow to brown plates, granules, or needles
6. Calcium oxalate: Various; dumbbell, octahedral, or envelope shapes
7. Leucine: Yellow to brown spheres, often with striations

ALKALINE URINE CRYSTALS AND THEIR APPEARANCE UNDER A MICROSCOPE

1. Triple phosphate: Triangular or hexagonal prisms, similar to a coffin shape
2. Calcium phosphate: Crystals may be irregularly-shaped and large, or in granular sheets or plates
3. Amorphous phosphate: Colorless granules
4. Ammonium biurate: Brown or yellow, with striations; may contain irregular projections
5. Calcium carbonate: Small and colorless, often dumbbell-shaped

MAPLE SYRUP URINE DISEASE

Individuals with the genetic metabolic disorder known as maple syrup urine disease have a natural deficiency of branched-chain keto acid decarboxylase, resulting in a diminished metabolism of valine, leucine, and isoleucine. The condition gets its name from the aroma emanating from the urine, breath, and skin of infants with the condition. This condition is most common in the Amish and Mennonite communities, and can be identified with a Guthrie bacterial inhibition test. If it is not treated, it can lead to intellectual disability, hypoglycemia, convulsions, and even death.

CEREBROSPINAL FLUID

Cerebrospinal fluid fulfills a number of functions in the human body. It removes waste products, supplies nutrients to the nervous system, and supports the brain and spinal column. The average human produces 20 mL of this substance every hour, and typically has between 140 and 170 mL at any given time. Normal cerebrospinal fluid is clear and colorless. If the fluid is cloudy, this may be due to meningitis or hemorrhage; if it is yellow, this may indicate an elevated level of bilirubin or protein.

Cerebrospinal fluid is collected as follows: a spinal tap, otherwise known as a lumbar puncture, is made either between the third and fourth or fourth and fifth lumbar vertebrae. Three tubes of fluid are removed: one for microbiological analysis; one for hematological analysis; and one for chemical and serological analysis.

SEMEN ANALYSIS

These are the parameters for a semen analysis: General color and clarity of the semen should be a grayish-white and translucent. The pH should be between 7.3 and 7.8, and the viscosity of the semen (the resistance of the semen to flow) should get a rating of one on a scale of one to four. The volume of the entire ejaculate should be between two and five milliliters. Coagulation and liquefaction should occur within 30 minutes of collecting the sample. The motility of the sperm, or the percentage of sperm present that are moving, should be about 60% or higher. The percentage of sperm that are moving forward (forward progression) should be at least 50% or higher. The sperm count should be a minimum of 40 million sperm per total ejaculate. At least 30% of the sperm present should have a normal morphology, with no double or deformed tails or heads.

COLLECTION OF SEMINAL FLUID

Before his semen may be collected for an infertility analysis, and a male must be abstinent for three days. Such a waiting period is not necessary before other laboratory tests. Semen is collected in a sterile container and cannot be obtained in the presence of condoms or spermicides. Semen is collected and stored at room temperature.

NORMAL RESULTS FROM A SEMEN ANALYSIS

In a typical semen analysis, the following characteristics are considered:

- Viscosity: rated from zero (very low) to four (very viscous)
- Volume: normal range is between two and 5 mL
- Color: milky is normal
- pH: normal range is between 7.2 and 7
- Sperm count: normal range is between 20 and 160 million sperm per milliliter
- Motility (degree to which sperm move forward): normal range is between 50 and 60%, or three or four on a scale of zero to four
- Shape of sperm: normal shape is one head and one straight tail

TYPES OF FECAL MATTER

1. Watery: indicates diarrhea
2. Ribbon-like: indicates bowel obstruction
3. Black/tarry: indicates bleeding in the gastrointestinal tract
4. Frothy, bulky, or yellow colored: indicates malabsorption syndrome, in which stool contains too much fat
5. Containing mucus: indicates colitis or inflammation of the intestinal wall

SYNOVIAL FLUID

Synovial fluid, also known as joint fluid, lubricates and cushions the joints and delivers nutrients to cartilage. Synovial fluid is thick and stringy, and should either be clear or light yellow. Infections, inflammations, and bleeding may affect the consistency and color of synovial fluid. Gout is indicated by crystals in the fluid. A typical analysis of synovial fluid includes an analysis of visual characteristics as well as a differential counts and Gram stain.

PKU

Phenylketonuria, otherwise known as PKU, is a metabolic disorder in which phenylalanine is not easily converted into tyrosine. This genetic disorder is often caused by a lack of the catalyzing enzyme hydroxylase. If this condition is not treated, it can result in intellectual disability. Infants born with PKU will have urine with a distinct odor. The smell is caused by an elevated level of ketones. Infants should be tested within their first day of life. There are a few different tests for PKU: ferric chloride strips and the Guthrie bacterial inhibition test are the most common methods.

REFRACTOMETER

Refractometers are used to measure fluid concentration by assessing light refraction through a prism. Refractometers vary in size and sophistication (simple handheld devices to more complex digital devices), so procedures may vary. Generally, the instrument is calibrated with water before the sample is tested. Testing:

- Turn on equipment.
- Clean prism with cotton ball and ethanol or according to manufacturer's guidelines.
- Place sample on prism or in sample well and secure prism.
- Look through the eyepiece, adjust as needed for manual equipment.
- Read results expressed in Brix (1 degree Brix = 1 g sucrose in 100 g solution), refractive index (degree to which the light is bent), and/or specific gravity. Digital equipment provides a read-out. Note: Tables are available that provide the refractive index for most common materials

Refractometers may be used to assess urine specific gravity, serum copper sulfate, and serum protein. Sample temperature must be maintained within a prescribed temperature range for some types of refractometers.

MANUAL TESTING

Bilirubin	Uncoagulated blood sample allowed to clot at room temperature and then centrifuged and supernatant separated immediately for examination. Direct: Dilute sample by mixing 1 mL with 4 mL saline. Label 2 tubes for direct bilirubin (DB) and serum blank (SB). Place 1 mL diluted serum and 2 mL 0.05 hydrochloric acid in each tube. Place 0.5 mL Diazo II reagent in DB and in exactly 60 seconds add 0.1 mL ascorbic acid, mix, and add 1.5 mL alkaline tartrate and read color results in 5-10 minutes. To tube SB, place 0.5 mL Diazo I reagent, 0.5 mL ascorbic acid, and 1.5 mL alkaline tartrate, and mix to use as serum blank.
Occult blood (gastric)	Sample is applied to paper reagent strip coated with guaiac, which changes color to blue in the presence of blood within 1 minute. The sample may also be applied to a slide (thin smear), which is examined microscopically.

BODY FLUID CYTOCENTRIFUGATION

Cytocentrifugation ("cytospin") uses a special centrifuge with slide holders that have attached funnels to hold body fluid that has been mixed with a medium in prescribed amounts. The process is able to concentrate cells that occur in small numbers in a sample. During centrifugation (usually at about 500 rpm for about 5 minutes), the fluid is wicked into a filter and onto a slide in a thin monolayer. Albumin (11% or 22%) may be added to serous fluids to preserve morphology as centrifugation may result in some distortion (although clumping patterns and ratio of nucleus to cytoplasm are unchanged). Albumin should not be added to synovial fluid. Cells in body fluids are similar to those in peripheral blood, and morphology is similar but counts are usually less. Once the slide is prepared, staining may be done to facilitate evaluation.

AMNIOTIC FLUID MEASUREMENTS

1. The lecithin/sphingomyelin ratio in the amniotic fluid is a good indicator for the lung maturity of the fetus. Via amniocentesis, a sample of surfactant in the amniotic fluid is removed. The lecithin/sphingomyelin ratio is then calculated. If the ratio is less than 2, then the fetal lungs are not producing enough surfactant, and this is an indicator that the fetal lungs may be immature (wet). Determining the lecithin/sphingomyelin ratio is very important because it can help predict and/or prevent fetal respiratory distress after birth.

2. The concentrations of creatinine and urea nitrogen in amniotic fluid are useful for helping determine if amniotic fluid is contaminated with any maternal urine. Using amniocentesis, a sample of amniotic fluid is extracted from the mother's uterus. Because creatinine and urea nitrogen concentrations in the mother's urine are much greater (on the order of ten to fifty times greater) than those concentrations in amniotic fluid, an unexpected high concentration of creatinine and/or urea nitrogen in the amniotic fluid can indicate contamination of the amniotic fluid with maternal urine, often by bladder puncture.

Practice Test

1. Receiving cannot accept a specimen unless it has

    a. A correct, legible label
    b. An uncontaminated, signed requisition with billing information
    c. An intact container with correct media
    d. All of the above

2. A laboratory refrigerator used to store volatile, flammable liquids can hold

    a. 120 gallons of class I, II, and IIIA liquids
    b. 180 gallons of class I, II, and IIIA liquids
    c. 200 gallons of class I, II, and IIIA liquids
    d. 50 gallons of class I, II, and IIIA liquids

3. Disease incidence predicts

    a. How probable it is a patient will develop a disease, and its etiology
    b. How likely a test result is to be right or wrong, given certain variables
    c. How likely the patient with a negative test really does not have the condition
    d. How likely the patient with a positive test result really has the condition

4. Beer's law in spectrophotometry

    a. Means a transparent sample transmits 0% light
    b. Only applies if absorbance is between 0.1 and 1.0
    c. Means an opaque sample transmits 100% light
    d. Uses a visible spectrum from 340 nm to 500 nm

5. Naming bacteria by looking at their size and shape under the microscope, and the colony morphology on media is

    a. Differential identification
    b. Numeric taxonomy
    c. Presumptive identification
    d. TaqMan electrophoresis

6. The hospital department that studies alcohol, drugs, poisons, and heavy metals is

    a. Serology/Immunology
    b. Toxicology
    c. Cytology
    d. Endocrinology

7. A hemoglobin electrophoresis result of adult hemoglobin (HbA) or HbA2 means the patient has

    a. Sickle cell anemia
    b. Fetal hemoglobin
    c. Normal hemoglobin
    d. Hemolytic anemia

8. US law overrides the patient's right to confidentiality if

a. The patient has a sexually transmitted disease or tuberculosis (TB).
b. The caregiver is likely to be infected.
c. Authorities suspect child abuse or neglect under CAPTA.
d. All of the above

9. The recall rate is also known as the

a. Sensitivity
b. Specificity
c. Aliquot
d. Circadian rhythm

10. Biochemistry usually requires

a. Lavender, light blue, and black blood collection tubes
b. Red, pink, and yellow blood collection tubes
c. Green, gray, and marbled serum-separator tube (SST) blood collection tubes
d. Navy, purple, and brown blood collection tubes

11. A normal kidney function study shows a

a. BUN to creatinine ratio between 15:1 and 20:1
b. Alkaline phosphatase 30 to 85 international milliunits/mL
c. Serum aspartate aminotransferase 5 to 40 international units/L
d. Amylase 56 to 190 international units/L

12. A newborn's jaundice could be caused by

a. Erythroblastosis fetalis
b. Kernicterus
c. Physiologic jaundice from poor fluid intake
d. All of the above

13. Lipids from carbohydrate and alcohol sources are

a. Anions
b. Triglycerides
c. Cholesterol
d. Eluent

14. When serum proteins indicate disease, the doctor usually follows up with

a. Total protein, albumin, and globulin
b. Ascites
c. Protein electrophoresis
d. Bilirubin

15. Elevated creatine phosphokinase (CPK) could mean myocardial infarction, but could also mean

a. Alcoholism, hypothyroidism, cardioversion, or clofibrate use
b. Aspirin, burns, warfarin, or sickle cell anemia
c. Lung disease or congestive heart failure
d. Crushing injury, bowel infarction, or opiate use

16. A patient whose cortisol level is high at both 8:00 AM and 4:00 PM likely has

    a. Addison's disease
    b. Natriuretic factor
    c. Diabetes insipidus
    d. Cushing syndrome

17. Decreased sodium in the blood is

    a. Hypernatremia, often from diabetes, burns, or Cushing syndrome
    b. Hyponatremia, often from vomiting and diarrhea, furosemide, or Addison's disease
    c. Hyperkalemia, often from acidosis, spironolactone, or kidney failure
    d. Hypokalemia, often from alkalosis, stomach cancer, or eating too much licorice

18. CPK in a patient with a myocardial infarction will

    a. Rise 6 hours after heart attack, peak in 18 hours, and return to baseline in 3 days
    b. Rise 6 to 10 hours after heart attack, peak at 12 to 48 hours, and return to baseline in 4 days
    c. Rise 24 to 72 hours after heart attack, peak in 4 days, and return to baseline in 14 days
    d. Cause a corresponding rise in alpha-fetoprotein

19. The panic value for blood pH is

    a. 7.35
    b. Less than 7.20
    c. 80 to 100 torr
    d. 4.0 to 8.0 mcg/L

20. When performing a sweat test for cystic fibrosis, the MT ensures

    a. The current never exceeds 4 mA for 5 min and 25 volts.
    b. The current is 10 mA for 30 min and 10 volts.
    c. The current does not pass the patient's trunk.
    d. Both a and c are correct

21. If the doctor suspects the patient has Hodgkin disease, then the correct stain for the smear is

    a. Periodic acid-Schiff (PAS)
    b. Sudan black B (SBB)
    c. Leukocyte alkaline phosphatase (LAP)
    d. Lactophenol cotton blue (LPCB)

22. A battlement scan is preferable to a wedge scan for studying bone marrow because

    a. Battlement technique distributes cells evenly across the slide.
    b. Lymphocytes concentrate in the feather.
    c. Wedge technique causes leukocytes to pool in different sections of the slide.
    d. Both a and c

23. A bleeding patient with a coagulation deficiency needs

    a. 225 mL of fresh frozen plasma at +18°C
    b. 15 mL of cryoprecipitate at +18°C
    c. 300 mL of platelet pheresis at +20°C
    d. 520 mL of whole blood at +4°C

24. **Confirm a fungal infection found through microscopy with a**

   a. Latex serology for cryptococcal antigen
   b. Fungal serology titer of more than 1:32 that increases x4 or more 3 weeks later
   c. Complement fixation for coccidiomycosis and histoplasmosis
   d. Immunodiffusion for blastomycosis.

25. **Two modern flocculation tests that replace the older Venereal Disease Research Laboratory (VDRL) test for syphilis screening are**

   a. Plasmacrit test (PCT) and rapid plasma reagin (RPR) test
   b. Fluorescent treponemal antibody absorption (FTA-ABS) and enzyme-linked immunosorbent assay (ELISA)
   c. Treponemal-specific microhemagglutination (MHA-TP) and T. pallidum particle agglutination test (TP-PA)
   d. Captia Syphilis-G enzyme immunoassay (EIA) and cold agglutinins

26. **To make a dilution of ½ or 1:2**

   a. Dilute ½ mL of serum with 2 mL of saline
   b. Dilute 1 mL of serum with 2 mL of saline
   c. Test undiluted serum for antibody/antigen reaction against a control
   d. Dilute 1 mL of serum with 1 mL of saline

27. **A Monospot test uses ingredients from**

   a. Guinea pig, cow, and horse
   b. Sheep, pig, and horse
   c. Dog, sheep, and rabbit
   d. Fish, cat, and ferret

28. **A prozone phenomenon occurs when performing an antibody titer on a patient with**

   a. Epstein-Barr virus (EBV)
   b. Raynaud disease
   c. Both syphilis and HIV
   d. Immunoglobulin G (IgG) antibodies

29. **An Rh- mother who is pregnant with the child of an Rh+ father needs Rh immunoglobulin (RhoGAM)**

   a. Even if the pregnancy ends in miscarriage or abortion
   b. At 6 to 28 weeks of pregnancy and again within 72 hours after her delivery.
   c. During her labor
   d. Both a and b

30. **If a patient has a mild transfusion reaction**

   a. Eosinophilia, hypocalcemia, leukopenia, and pancytopenia may occur.
   b. Dyscrasia, leukocytosis, hypercalcemia, and leukemia may occur.
   c. Anemia, hypokalemia, glycosuria, and pancytopenia may occur.
   d. Hemolysis, hyperkalemia, hypoglycemia, and hemoglobinuria may occur.

31. Type O blood has

    a. B antigen and anti-A antibody
    b. A antigen and anti-B antibody
    c. No A or B antigens and both anti-A and anti-B antibodies
    d. Both A and B antigens and no anti-A or anti-B antibodies

32. Choose the top priority transfusion patient from the following list.

    a. Cardiac surgery patient who lost more than 1,200 mL of blood
    b. Trauma patient with a hemoglobin of 5 g/dL
    c. Pernicious anemia patient
    d. Hemophiliac boy at regular clinic visit

33. Reject a transfusion request when

    a. Recipient blood specimen is hemolyzed.
    b. The patient armband does not have a unique identifier.
    c. Donor blood is lipemic, clotted, or contains foreign objects.
    d. All of the above

34. The continuous recording thermometer in a Blood Bank refrigerator must be set at

    a. +4°C
    b. 0°C
    c. +6°C
    d. -5°C

35. If the surgical team suspects the patient will hemorrhage, they order

    a. Frozen platelets
    b. Whole blood
    c. Factor VIII
    d. O-

36. When blood typing by hemagglutination, the last O-shape is in the #64 incubation well, before the blood becomes solid red dots. Report the titer as

    a. 1:128
    b. 1:64
    c. 1:1024
    d. 1:512

37. When using an automatic pipette to perform immunoassays, the laboratory must have a procedure in place to detect

    a. Assay signal response
    b. Target analytes
    c. Sensitivity validation
    d. Carryover effects

38. When gamma and scintillation counters are used for radioimmunoassay (RIA), each day the technologist must

    a. Calibrate, record the results, and compare them to the previous day's values

    b. Test the background radioactivity in multiwell counters only

    c. Lengthen the counting times for quantitative procedures to improve validity

    d. Decontaminate sinks and benches monthly

39. To diagnose a urinary tract infection correctly, the microbiology lab requires a

    a. Midstream urine collection (MSU)

    b. Witnessed urine collection

    c. 24-hour urine collection

    d. Random urine collection

40. When assisting the doctor with cerebrospinal fluid (CSF) collection, you need 4 tubes for

    a. Cell count, glucose and protein, gram stain and culture, virology/mycology/cytology.

    b. Immunoelectrophoresis

    c. Fungus, oncology, and SMA-12

    d. Neutrophilia, lymphocytophilia, glutamine, and lactate dehydrogenase (LDH)

41. Fusobacteria cause

    a. Botulism and Listeria infections

    b. Lyme disease and Helicobacter pylori stomach ulcers

    c. Pyorrhea and Lemierre syndrome

    d. Chlamydial genital infections and pneumonia

42. The type of media required to incubate a TB culture correctly is

    a. Tinsdale

    b. Sheep blood agar

    c. Modified Wadowsky-Yee (MWY)

    d. Löwenstein-Jensen (LJ) egg

43. To find parasites under the microscope, set the magnification to

    a. 40x

    b. 10x

    c. 1,000x

    d. 400x

44. Identify the parasite that must be reported to Public Health authorities

    a. Crypto (Cryptosporidium parvum)

    b. Hookworm (Ancylostoma duodenale)

    c. Tapeworm (Cestoda)

    d. Pinworm (Enterobius)

45. To identify motile trophozoites

    a. Examine blood smears and blood antigens

    b. Perform a string test

    c. Use Snap n' Stain on sputum

    d. Wet mount fresh, liquid stool with LPCB stain

46. **Public Health requires you to keep positive parasitology samples preserved for**

    a. The patient's lifetime
    b. One year
    c. Ten years
    d. One month

47. **Shine a Wood's lamp over the patient's skin to help you collect**

    a. Malaria specimens
    b. Public Health specimens
    c. Toxicology specimens
    d. Mycology specimens

48. **When the doctor orders acid-fast stain to detect TB, the technologist**

    a. Looks for red bacteria under the oil-immersion lens
    b. Lyzes the cells by holding them in a Bunsen burner flame 30 seconds
    c. Pours 1% methylene blue stain into the LJ egg plate
    d. Decolorizes the bacteria with acetone and water solution

49. **Normal urinary output for a 24-hour urine test is**

    a. 4 quarts
    b. 150 to 500 mL
    c. 30 L
    d. 750 to 2,000 mL

50. **Urate crystals found during microscopic urinalysis indicate**

    a. Urea-splitting bacteria are present
    b. Poisoning
    c. Gout
    d. Hyperparathyroidism

Answer Key and Explanations

Question	Question	Question	Question	Question
1. D	11. A	21. C	31. C	41. C
2. A	12. D	22. D	32. B	42. D
3. A	13. B	23. A	33. D	43. B
4. B	14. C	24. B	34. A	44. A
5. C	15. A	25. A	35. A	45. D
6. B	16. D	26. D	36. B	46. B
7. C	17. B	27. A	37. D	47. D
8. D	18. A	28. C	38. A	48. A
9. A	19. B	29. D	39. A	49. D
10. C	20. D	30. A	40. A	50. C

Answer Explanations

1. D: Receiving cannot accession a specimen without

- A label that clearly states the patient's name, collection date, doctor's name and contact information, specimen type, and test required.
- An uncontaminated, valid requisition bearing the doctor's signature, patient's billing information, and pertinent information (acute or convalescent phase, antibiotic use, fever, or traveler).
- Intact specimen container.
- Correct media type or preservative used for the specimen type.
- Same-day collection date, or preincubated at room temperature or subcultivated, and then vented, to prevent false-negatives of nonfermentative species.

If the specimen does not meet these conditions, call the doctor's office and get the missing information. Discard the specimen if you cannot obtain full information, and inform the doctor's office that recollection is required.

2. A: Class IA, IB, and IC are flammables. Class II, IIIA, and IIIB are combustibles. No more than 120 gallons of class I, II, and IIIA liquids can be stored in a lab fridge, and, of those, no more than 60 gallons may be class I and II. Do not locate more than three storage cabinets in one fire area. No more than 50% of the flammables can be stored for teaching. Use DOT-approved glass, metal, or polyethylene containers no larger than 1.1 gallons (4 liters).

3. A: because disease incidence measures how prevalent a disease is among a given population in a specific place, over a specific time. Incidence predicts how probable it is a patient will develop a disease, and its etiology (likely cause). B, C, and D are incorrect because they refer to a related concept called predicted values, which estimate how likely a test result is to be right or wrong, given certain variables such as the patient's age, occupation, race, income, how long the symptoms have lasted, and if there is fever.

4. B: because Beer's law states absorbance is proportional to the concentration of a solution, but Beer's law only applies if absorbance is between 0.1 and 1.0. Different substances absorb different light wavelengths, so a spectrophotometer (Spec-20) compares the intensity of light entering a sample and exiting from it (percent transmittance) to find the concentration of the sample. A completely transparent sample has 100% transmittance. A completely opaque sample has 0% transmittance. Visible spectrum light ranges from 440 nm to 700 nm.

5. C: Note the color, outline (circular, rhizoid, or wavy), elevation (convex, flat, or raised), and translucency (opaque, translucent, or transparent) for presumptive identification. Differential identification means naming bacteria according to their headspace gases and volatile compounds they release as they grow on media, with a spectrometer (microDMx). Adanson's numerical taxonomy (phonetics) ranks microorganisms according to how similar they are genetically and morphologically. Closely related bacteria form a cluster, which is classified into objective, repeatable taxa. TaqMan, SWOrRD, and MicroSeq are quick screening kits. They are not as accurate as cultures but are quicker when time is critical. Polymerase chain reaction (PCR) in quick kits amplifies the genetic material, and then the 1450 base pair region of the 16S rDNA gene is sequenced by electrophoresis.

6. B: Serology/Immunology studies antibodies in the liquid part of blood. Cytology studies cells for cancer, such as Pap smears. Endocrinology studies hormones, such as diabetes and acromegaly.

7. C: Hemoglobin electrophoresis differentiates hemoglobin into normal HbA and normal HbA2, or abnormal HbS in sickle cell patients, or HbC in hemolytic anemia patients, or HbF in a fetus or newborn.

8. D: Doctors, nurses, social workers, chiropractors, law officers, daycare staff, clergy, teachers, and psychologists were declared mandatory reporters in 1996. This means they must report certain occurrences or suspicions orally to the proper authorities within 24 hours and follow up with a written report within 48 hours. For example, a doctor must report STD or TB to Public Health to prevent an epidemic. Caregivers have the right to know the patient's diagnosis if it puts them at risk for infection or assault. Suspicion of child abuse, exploitation, or neglect is reported to Child Protective Services under the Child Abuse Prevention and Treatment Act (CAPTA). Each state has an abuse hotline. Many states require anyone who has reasonable cause to report child or elder abuse or face civil liability. You must know the law of the state in which you practice.

9. A: Sensitivity (recall rate) measures how many times a test produces true-positive results, which indicates a patient probably has a disease, compared with the gold standard test for that particular illness. Sensitivity allows early detection of disease and prevents epidemics. Divide the number of patients who definitely have the disease and test positive by the total patients tested who have the disease (including those who tested false-negative), and multiply by 100 to obtain the percentage sensitivity. Specificity measures how many times a test produces true-negative results, meaning patients probably do not have a disease, compared with the gold standard test for that particular illness. Specificity is important for cancer chemotherapy and other toxic treatments. Aliquot is dividing a solution into equal parts. Aliquot allows very expensive reagents or drugs, and blood samples that are below scale, to be used efficiently. Circadian rhythm is a normal daily flow that affects hormones, which are normally higher in the morning than in the afternoon.

10. C: Hematology requires mostly lavender, light blue, and black tubes. Blood Bank and Public Health require red, pink, and yellow tubes. Toxicology requires navy, purple, and brown tubes. If you draw the wrong color tube, it contains an inappropriate anticoagulant, and the test will be invalidated.

11. A: Blood urea nitrogen (BUN) and creatinine are waste products of protein metabolism, measured in kidney function tests performed with a 24-hour urine. If the kidneys do not filter properly, creatinine output in the urine decreases, and creatine blood levels increase. High creatinine (more than 1.5 mg/dL) and BUN (more than 20 mg/dL) means the patient has a kidney disease (e.g., glomerulonephritis, pyelonephritis, stones, tubular necrosis, tumors). BUN and creatinine must be in correct proportion for optimal health. ALP and AST are liver function tests. Amylase is a pancreas test.

12. D: Newborn jaundice is different from adult jaundice. Babies have more red blood cells and reticulocytes than adults do. Babies have immature livers that are not yet efficient at breaking down bilirubin. Adult jaundice is usually from hepatitis or cirrhosis of the liver. Erythroblastosis fetalis means the baby's Rh factor is incompatible with his mother's Rh, leading to hemolytic disease of the newborn. Kernicterus means the bilirubin is greater than 5 mg/dL, resulting in hemolytic anemia if not treated with phototherapy (blue lights). Physiologic jaundice occurs in breastfed babies released from the hospital too early and without a vitamin K injection, but resolves in a week with adequate fluids.

13. B: Anions are negatively charged ions of chloride and bicarbonate. Cholesterol is lipids from animal sources that climb after a fatty meal. An eluent is a solvent used for chromatography.

14. C: The serum proteins test includes total protein, albumin, and globulin. Ascites is swelling of the abdomen from extra fluid in the peritoneum, resulting from end-stage diseases of the heart, kidney, liver, ovary, and pancreas. When serum proteins make the doctor suspect one of these diseases, the doctor follows up with protein electrophoresis. Four globulin fractionations are added to the total protein and albumin alpha-1 globulin, alpha-2 globulin, beta globulin, and gamma globulin. Electrophoresis patterns and the patient's history of drug use help pinpoint the diagnosis, which may extend to rheumatoid arthritis, muscle tumors, and immune deficiencies. Bilirubin is the brownish-red bile pigment from broken down blood cells in the liver.

15. A: Cardiac enzymes elevate soon after a heart attack, but that is not the only possible root cause. CPK elevates in alcoholism; cardiac catheterization; stroke; clofibrate use; electric shock applied during resuscitation; low thyroid hormone and high thyroid stimulating hormone; and after surgery. B and D refer to situations that cause AST enzyme to rise. C refers to situations that cause LDH enzyme to rise.

16. D: Cortisol is an adrenal stress hormone that is normally higher around 800 in the morning (6 to 28 mcg/dL) and lower at 400 in the afternoon (2 to 12 mcg/dL). The fluctuation is a normal diurnal variation. Cushing syndrome patients have sustained high cortisol. Addison's disease patients have chronically low cortisol levels, diagnosed by a 24-hour urine test for 17-hydroxycorticosteroids. Abnormal cortisol levels also appear in thyroid and pituitary gland disease, obesity, and cancer, and when steroids, diuretics, or birth control pills are used, but it is not the same pattern as Cushing syndrome. B refers to atrial natriuretic factor (ANF), produced by the heart's atria during volume overload and high blood pressure.

17. B: Hyponatremia results from too much water and not enough salt in the bloodstream. Hyponatremia often presents as a urine sample with a specific gravity (SG) lower than the normal 1.015 to 1.025 and closer to the SG of water (1.000). Hypernatremia refers to too much salt in the bloodstream, which increases SG above 1.025. Hyperkalemia and hypokalemia refer to the level of potassium, not sodium.

18. A: CPK is the first enzyme to rise following a heart attack, so doctors measure it before the other cardiac enzymes. If creatine kinase-MB (CK-MB) rises, it means the heart sustained severe damage. B refers to the response of AST to a heart attack. C refers to the response of LDH to a heart attack. D does not apply because alpha-fetoprotein (AFP) is used to find liver disease, testicular cancer, and birth defects.

19. B: pH stands for percentage of hydrogen. A blood pH test is performed with arterial blood gasses to determine if the patient has acidosis or alkalosis. The blood must be kept in a narrow range of pH from 7.35 to 7.45, so answer A would be low normal. Answer C, 80 to 100 torr, refers to normal percentage of oxygen. D is incorrect because an abnormal PSA result for prostate cancer is unrelated to blood pH.

20. D: When performing a sweat test for cystic fibrosis, the technologist must avoid burning the patient or causing depolarization of the heart. The technologist uses only a battery-powered iontophoretic current and it cannot exceed 4 mA for 5 minutes. The technologist uses only the patient's arm or leg for sweat collection and ensures the electrodes do not cross over the patient's trunk. The technologist never performs iontophoresis near an open oxygen source, but asks the nurse to give the patient a face mask or nasal cannula during the test.

21. C: Hematologists use LAP stain to highlight neutrophils when the patient has many white blood cells but not leukemia (leukemic reaction). Microbiologists use periodic acid-Schiff (PAS) to stain carbohydrates, collagen, fibrin, and mucin purple. Sudan black B (SBB) is specifically for acute leukemia patients; it helps to differentiate between immature cells by staining lipids in myeloid leukemia that are absent in lymphoid leukemia. LPCB is mixed with 10% potassium hydroxide (KOH) to identify fungus.

22. D: Make a bone marrow slide with a battlement technique so the review is standardized, with even cell distribution. Wedge push technique (feathered end) causes the white cells to pool unevenly on the slide. On the side edges and in the feather of a wedge push slide, concentrated pockets of eosinophils, monocytes, and segmented neutrophils will be found. Small lymphocytes concentrate in the center of the slide.

23. A: Fresh frozen plasma can be used for a bleeding patient with a coagulation deficiency, or a trauma patient who needs additional red blood cells. Reserve whole blood for the resuscitation of trauma victims. Cryoprecipitate is appropriate for hemophiliacs, von Willebrand disease, and hypofibrinogenemia. Platelet pheresis is useful for patients with thrombocytopenia or platelet dysfunction.

24. B: First, gently scrape suspected fungus off the patient's skin. Mix two drops of 10% potassium hydroxide (KOH) and one drop of LPCB on a glass slide, cover it, and warm it to observe budding yeasts. Add a drop of calcofluor white before warming to see fluorescent infected tissue. Put a drop of India ink on a wet mount to see clear cryptococcal capsules. Confirm the microscopic exam with fungal serology when you test the skin scraping and again in three weeks. The doctor may follow up by ordering latex serology for cryptococcal antigen to find meningitis, complement fixation for coccidiomycosis and histoplasmosis, and immunodiffusion for blastomycosis.

25. A: The old screening test for syphilis is VDRL, which measures Treponema pallidum antibodies by flocculation reaction to the diphosphatidyl glycerol in ox heart extract. However, VDRL misses cases of syphilis that are less than four weeks old, and half of cases that are in the late stages. VDRL is not very sensitive, and often gives a false-positive result for patients with the following conditions pregnancy, hepatitis, HIV, leprosy, lupus (SLE), Lyme disease, malaria, mononucleosis, pneumonia, rheumatic fever, or rheumatoid arthritis. PCT and RCR are less likely to be confounded, and since they require less blood, are replacing VDRL. ELISA confirms syphilis infection by identifying the specific antibodies. FTA-ABS is 100% accurate for secondary syphilis, but it is expensive, and the patient will always test positive once infected. Captia is required to confirm RPR. Cold agglutinins increase in children with congenital syphilis.

26. D: You must know how to dilute to perform a titer, which measures how many times a blood sample must be diluted with saline before an antibody can no longer be found in it.

First, check the antibody/antigen reaction against the controls with undiluted serum. To prevent blood clotting (rouleaux formation) during dilution, warm the blood and saline to body temperature (37°C) for 10 minutes before diluting. Dilute 1 mL of serum with 1 mL of saline for a dilution of ½, or 12. Pipette off 1 mL of this dilution into an aliquot tube. Add 1 mL of saline, and it becomes a 14 dilution. If you dilute up to 132 and get no reaction, the end-point titer is 16.

27. A: Monospot heterophile antibodies test confirms an early infection of mononucleosis, caused by Epstein-Barr virus. If the infection is older than 9 weeks, then the doctor orders EBV antibody test. On a glass slide, mix a drop of the patient's blood with guinea pig kidney antigen to absorb Forssman antibodies. Add beef red blood stroma to absorb non-Forssman antibodies. Mix with horse blood. Guinea pig agglutination means the patient has early mononucleosis. Beef should not agglutinate. Monospot can be false-negative on children younger than 10, or before two weeks of infection. B, C, and D are not applicable to Monospot.

28. C: Patients coinfected with HIV and syphilis are immunosuppressed. When performing a titer to find antibodies in an HIV/syphilitic, beware prozone phenomenon. The coinfected patient's undiluted serum may produce a false-negative result because it does not agglutinate. Alternatively, it may show very little agglutination at low dilutions, but agglutinates more at higher dilutions because of excess antibodies. Monospot is used to find EBV mononucleosis. Reynaud disease is characterized by rouleaux formation and high cold agglutinin titers. IgG occurs in patients who are convalescing from mononucleosis.

29. D: RhoGAM is the brand name for Rh immunoglobulin. It is administered to Rh- women who acquired anti-D antibodies from a previous blood transfusion or pregnancy. The infant and father do not receive RhoGAM at all. If there is a live birth, the mother gets 300 mcg of RhoGAM during week 26 to 28 of her pregnancy, and again before her infant is 3 days old. If the pregnancy miscarries before week 13 or is aborted, then the mother gets a lower dose of 50 mcg of MICRhoGAM. If the miscarriage or abortion happens after week 13, use RhoGAM.

30. A: The first lab sign of a mild transfusion reaction is the oxyhemoglobin dissociation curve shifts left. Later, the number of eosinophils will increase and the calcium level will drop. Finally, white blood cells will decrease, and then all blood cells will decrease. Minimize the chance of transfusion reaction by washing the donor's red blood cells in sterile normal saline before transfusion. If the doctor anticipates a mild transfusion reaction, he/she may give antihistamines to the patient before transfusion, and may order the removal of white cells from the bag of blood by a Sepacell R-500 leukocyte reduction filter. Irradiated blood products prevent fatal transfusion-associated graft-versus-host disease (TA-GVHD). The safest way for a patient to prepare for elective surgery is to bank his own blood for transfusion (autologous donation).

31. C: No A or B antigens and both anti-A and anti-B antibodies. Type O- blood is the universal donor because it has no A or B antigens, or Rh+ antibodies. If there is no time to crossmatch a trauma patient, then O– blood is given without compatibility testing to prevent death. A routine type and cross takes 45 minutes and the delay could be fatal.

32.B: Blood Bank triages patients in the following priority sequence (1) emergency trauma victims with isovolemic anemia from hemorrhage; (2) surgical patients who lose more than 3 cups of blood; (3) regular users of coagulation factors. If you anticipate a blood shortage because of a massive trauma, then contact the nurse manager as soon as possible. The surgical team may decide to cancel elective surgery, or delay it until the patient is medically treated to reduce anemia. If surgery must proceed, the surgical team may consider the following blood conservation methods if you warn them ahead of time erythropoietin, autologous donations, or hemodilution before surgery; cell savers, hypotension, electrocautery, and lasers during surgery; and administration of antifibrinolytics after surgery.

33. D: A type and cross is very time-consuming (45 minutes) and must meet very specific safety standards to avoid a transfusion reaction. All of the following conditions must be met

- Specimens labeled at the patient's bedside with full name or the emergency department identification number; initials are unacceptable. Specimens must not have pink serum. Donor blood must not be clotted, fatty, or contaminated.

- Patient wears an identification band, which is checked at collection and transfusion times. The band must not be taped to the bed. The patient's name and a unique identification number (Blood Bank identification number, hospital number, health insurance number, or unique lifetime identifier) must appear on the band, in case there is a patient with a similar name.
- Requisitions must bear the collector's and identifier's names, collection date and time (in case antibodies develop), the ordering doctor's name, the amount and type of blood requested, the patient's date of birth (if known), relevant patient history (e.g., pregnant and bleeding; signs of transfusion reaction).

34. A: Other laboratory refrigerators can safely range from 0ºC to +6ºC. However, Blood Bank must keep blood products at a stable +4ºC to ensure their safety. Only freezers should be in the minus degrees range, as ice cr

35. A: The surgical team carefully reviews the patient's pre-op blood work to anticipate any complications that might occur in the operating room. An anesthetized patient whose heart rate increases during surgery, or whose blood pressure drops, can quickly lose 1.5 liters of blood. Initially, the surgical team will want frozen platelets standing by from Blood Bank. The nurses weigh the patient and count the number of saturated pads in the theater to help the surgeon and anesthetist calculate blood loss. A 2x2 gauze pad holds 5 mL of blood and a 4x4 gauze pad holds 12 mL of blood. If the blood loss approaches 500 mL, the surgeon orders a transfusion. Although plasma volume increases after blood loss, red cell volume does not return to normal for several weeks without compensation from a transfusion. Whole blood may be required to ensure recovery is as quick and painless as possible.

36. B: Blood typing (A, B, O) to prevent blood transfusion reactions is usually performed by hemagglutination. Antibodies crosslink red blood cells coated with antigen. Nonagglutinated blood forms a solid red dot at the bottom of an incubation well. Agglutinated blood appears diffuse or O-shaped at the bottom of an incubation well. The technologist makes serial dilutions of serum in incubation wells and measures the highest dilution still capable of agglutinating the blood. Most agglutination reactions occur in less than 2 minutes. Label the control wells Neg and Pos. Label the remaining incubation wells 2, 4, 8, 16, 32, 64, 128, 256, 512, and 1024 for the serial dilutions. Look along the row of wells for the last O-shape before the blood becomes solid red dots. If the last O is at 64, then report the titer as 1:64.

37. D: If the laboratory's immunoassay setup includes an automatic pipette, then the lab manager must create a procedure to determine if carryover effects are contaminating the samples. The most common procedure requires running known high samples first, followed by known low samples. If the results of the low-level material are affected, then carryover is present. The procedure must define the benchmark below which low-level samples are affected. Quality Assurance must review the results of each analytical run to ensure there are no results exceeding the benchmark. The procedure then states what the technologist must do with the subsequent samples. Usually, the technologist is expected to repeat the subsequent samples, using a clean pipette for each.

38. A: The technologist must determine if the machines are performing to the standard with daily radioisotope calibrations that are recorded for accreditation purposes. Sinks and benches are decontaminated daily, not monthly. If the lab uses or stores radionuclides in excess of those found in commercial 125-I RIA kits, then the Nuclear Regulatory Commission requires the technologist to be familiar with the radiation manual, which covers safe shielding, storage, decontamination, counting, disposal, and reporting procedures.

39. A: MSU is required to diagnose cystitis and pyelitis accurately. Witnessed collection is only required for drug testing. 24-hour urines are for hormone tests. Random urine may have contamination, so while it is suitable for chemistry, random urine is inaccurate for microbiology. Collect midstream urine any time of day, in a sterile, lidded container. Your microbiologist may want the patient to use a benzalkonium chloride wipe before collection. Without a wipe, the sample is not a clean catch. Do not touch the inside of the container, as it contaminates the specimen and produces a false-positive.

40. A: Only a physician can collect cerebrospinal fluid (CSF) from a lumbar puncture. The medical technologist just prepares a collection tray and assists as ordered. The tray must contain the following iodine prep; alcohol prep; 3 cc of 1% lidocaine; 25g, 5/8" needle; 22g, 1.5" needle; atraumatic spinal needle (to prevent postcollection headache); syringe; four sterile red stoppered tubes; 4x4 gauze; sponge forceps; sterile towels; small basin; and a Band-Aid. The physician collects the fluid between L3 and L4 in the patient's spine and hands you the tubes. Label one tube each for cell count, glucose and protein, gram stain and culture, and virology/mycology/cytology. You only need a fifth tube if the physician wants globulin immunoelectrophoresis, which is rare. C and D tests are included in A, and it is unnecessary to requisition them separately.

41. C: The pathogenic phyla are xenobacteria, cyanobacteria, firmicutes, flavobacteria, fusobacteria, planctomycetes, proteobacteria, spirochaetes, and verrucomicrobia. Planctomycetes causes chlamydia and pneumonia. Spirochaetes cause Lyme disease. Proteobacteria causes stomach ulcers. Firmicutes cause food poisoning. Fusobacteria cause pockets of pus in the gums that can break off into septic blood clots in the jugular vein of the neck. The septic clots can travel to cause abscesses in distant parts of the body, such as the brain, joints, kidney, and liver. Lemierre syndrome from gum disease was common until the discovery of antibiotics.

42. D: Tuberculosis is a fussy bacterium to grow in the lab and requires egg media. Tinsdale is used to find C. diphtheria. Sheep blood is used to find slow-growing anaerobic bacteria. MYW is used to find Legionella pneumonia. It is important for the medical technologist to know what type of infection the doctor suspects, so the correct media can be used for culture. Failure to pick the correct media may result in a false-negative and the disease will go undiagnosed.

43. B: To find parasites such as worms, set the microscope's magnification to 10x. Parasites often cause bleeding, so set the microscope to 40x to find the blood cells. Higher powers are unnecessary to view animal parasites and count cells, and would just slow down the medical technologist's slide reading. Calibrate the ocular micrometer every time a new technologist is hired, each time you change optics, and annually thereafter.

44. A: In the United States, the medical technologist is required by law to report the following nine parasites to Public Health authorities if they are found in patient samples Cryptosporidium parvum, Cyclospora cayetanensis, Entamoeba histolytica, hematoxylin, Giardia duodenalis, Plasmodium falciparum, Taenia, Trichinella spiralis, and Enterobius vermicularis. Hookworm, tapeworm, and pinworm are very common infestations and do not need to be reported. Your lab must provide reference slides or a parasite atlas for you to compare against the patients' specimens. Keep positive specimens in your lab for at least one year, either as a permanently stained slide, or as a preserved stool sample that is safely stored. Public Health may order them for examination.

45. D: Giardia lamblia is a parasite that lives in the small intestine of humans who consume contaminated food or water. Giardia causes traveler's diarrhea. Giardia cysts are activated by stomach acid and become trophozoites. The medical technologist can get the patient to swallow a string for several hours and then examine it for trophozoites, but many patients are uncooperative and prefer to leave a stool sample instead. To prepare the wet mount, strain well-formed stool. Concentrate it in the centrifuge at 2000 rpm for 4 minutes in a conical tube. Ream the tube with a wooden stick. Add 10% formalin. Make a tan suspension. You should be able to read a newspaper through the slide. Examine microscopically at 10x for parasites and 40x for blood. Use an ocular micrometer to measure parasites. Mix stool with PVA plastic powder to glue it onto the slide before permanent staining with iodine or Snap n' Stain.

46. B: Parasites are a serious Public Health issue. It is important to prevent parasites acquired in foreign countries from spreading through the American populace. Even though you check your patient's specimen against reference slides or a parasite atlas, you could miss rare species or misidentify the parasite in its different stages of development. A Public Health official has the right to check your slide for one year after initial testing. To ensure your test is accurate, use positive and negative controls to check your antigens every time you receive a new shipment and every month thereafter. Use the right stain for the right specimen. Refrigerate stool within three hours of receiving it, if you do not have time to fix it with preservative.

47. D: The medical technologist uses a Wood's lamp to help identify fungus on the patient's skin before collecting it. Fungus will fluoresce bright lime green under the Wood's light, so the medical technologist will find it easily and can scrape it off with a tongue depressor into a sterile container for testing. Malaria parasites are found in blood smears. Public Health specimens are usually blood serology or stool for parasites. Toxicology specimens are usually red, navy, or purple stoppered blood tubes for drugs or heavy metals.

48. A: The technologist submerges the TB smear for five minutes in Kinyoun carbol fuchsin stain, decolorizes with a 70% ethanol/0.5% hydrochloric acid solution, followed by 1% methylene blue stain for 1 minute. Tubercle bacteria appear red under the oil-immersion lens. Do not hold the slide in the flame. It lyzes the cells by cooking them. If the slide feels too hot when placed on the back of your hand, then heat killed the TB bacteria. Do not overwash with water, and do not use acetone to decolorize.

49. D: A patient should produce at least 500 mL (2 cups) of urine every day. Ideally, a patient should produce 750 mL (3 cups) to 2,000 mL (5 cups) of urine to maintain good health. If the patient has vomiting and diarrhea, or an enlarged prostate gland or severe infection, or uses too much medication, then he will produce scanty urine (oliguria). Some of the drug overdoses that decrease urinary output are anticholinergics, methotrexate, and diuretics. Patients whose kidneys are failing have anuria, which strictly interpreted means absence of urine, but they actually produce 100 mL or less of urine per day. Patients who have diabetes insipidus or diabetes mellitus often produce far too much urine (3½ quarts or more). They are very thirsty and may drink more than a gallon of fluid per day (more than 12 glasses). The antidepressant lithium is one drug that can cause frequent urination as an adverse effect.

50. C: Patients with gout have extreme pain in their great toes due to needles of uric acid crystals that form around their joints. Patients with struvite crystals in their urine have bacterial infections. Patients with tyrosine or cystine crystals in their urine may be poisoned or have a serious metabolic disorder. Patients with phosphate or calcium oxalate crystals in their urine have too much parathyroid hormone or malabsorption. Crystals do not appear in healthy urine.

How to Overcome Test Anxiety

Just the thought of taking a test is enough to make most people a little nervous. A test is an important event that can have a long-term impact on your future, so it's important to take it seriously and it's natural to feel anxious about performing well. But just because anxiety is normal, that doesn't mean that it's helpful in test taking, or that you should simply accept it as part of your life. Anxiety can have a variety of effects. These effects can be mild, like making you feel slightly nervous, or severe, like blocking your ability to focus or remember even a simple detail.

If you experience test anxiety—whether severe or mild—it's important to know how to beat it. To discover this, first you need to understand what causes test anxiety.

Causes of Test Anxiety

While we often think of anxiety as an uncontrollable emotional state, it can actually be caused by simple, practical things. One of the most common causes of test anxiety is that a person does not feel adequately prepared for their test. This feeling can be the result of many different issues such as poor study habits or lack of organization, but the most common culprit is time management. Starting to study too late, failing to organize your study time to cover all of the material, or being distracted while you study will mean that you're not well prepared for the test. This may lead to cramming the night before, which will cause you to be physically and mentally exhausted for the test. Poor time management also contributes to feelings of stress, fear, and hopelessness as you realize you are not well prepared but don't know what to do about it.

Other times, test anxiety is not related to your preparation for the test but comes from unresolved fear. This may be a past failure on a test, or poor performance on tests in general. It may come from comparing yourself to others who seem to be performing better or from the stress of living up to expectations. Anxiety may be driven by fears of the future—how failure on this test would affect your educational and career goals. These fears are often completely irrational, but they can still negatively impact your test performance.

> **Review Video: 3 Reasons You Have Test Anxiety**
> Visit mometrix.com/academy and enter code: 428468

Elements of Test Anxiety

As mentioned earlier, test anxiety is considered to be an emotional state, but it has physical and mental components as well. Sometimes you may not even realize that you are suffering from test anxiety until you notice the physical symptoms. These can include trembling hands, rapid heartbeat, sweating, nausea, and tense muscles. Extreme anxiety may lead to fainting or vomiting. Obviously, any of these symptoms can have a negative impact on testing. It is important to recognize them as soon as they begin to occur so that you can address the problem before it damages your performance.

> **Review Video: 3 Ways to Tell You Have Test Anxiety**
> Visit mometrix.com/academy and enter code: 927847

The mental components of test anxiety include trouble focusing and inability to remember learned information. During a test, your mind is on high alert, which can help you recall information and stay focused for an extended period of time. However, anxiety interferes with your mind's natural processes, causing you to blank out, even on the questions you know well. The strain of testing during anxiety makes it difficult to stay focused, especially on a test that may take several hours. Extreme anxiety can take a huge mental toll, making it difficult not only to recall test information but even to understand the test questions or pull your thoughts together.

> **Review Video: How Test Anxiety Affects Memory**
> Visit mometrix.com/academy and enter code: 609003

Effects of Test Anxiety

Test anxiety is like a disease—if left untreated, it will get progressively worse. Anxiety leads to poor performance, and this reinforces the feelings of fear and failure, which in turn lead to poor performances on subsequent tests. It can grow from a mild nervousness to a crippling condition. If allowed to progress, test anxiety can have a big impact on your schooling, and consequently on your future.

Test anxiety can spread to other parts of your life. Anxiety on tests can become anxiety in any stressful situation, and blanking on a test can turn into panicking in a job situation. But fortunately, you don't have to let anxiety rule your testing and determine your grades. There are a number of relatively simple steps you can take to move past anxiety and function normally on a test and in the rest of life.

> **Review Video: How Test Anxiety Impacts Your Grades**
> Visit mometrix.com/academy and enter code: 939819

Physical Steps for Beating Test Anxiety

While test anxiety is a serious problem, the good news is that it can be overcome. It doesn't have to control your ability to think and remember information. While it may take time, you can begin taking steps today to beat anxiety.

Just as your first hint that you may be struggling with anxiety comes from the physical symptoms, the first step to treating it is also physical. Rest is crucial for having a clear, strong mind. If you are tired, it is much easier to give in to anxiety. But if you establish good sleep habits, your body and mind will be ready to perform optimally, without the strain of exhaustion. Additionally, sleeping well helps you to retain information better, so you're more likely to recall the answers when you see the test questions.

Getting good sleep means more than going to bed on time. It's important to allow your brain time to relax. Take study breaks from time to time so it doesn't get overworked, and don't study right before bed. Take time to rest your mind before trying to rest your body, or you may find it difficult to fall asleep.

> **Review Video: <u>The Importance of Sleep for Your Brain</u>**
> Visit mometrix.com/academy and enter code: 319338

Along with sleep, other aspects of physical health are important in preparing for a test. Good nutrition is vital for good brain function. Sugary foods and drinks may give a burst of energy but this burst is followed by a crash, both physically and emotionally. Instead, fuel your body with protein and vitamin-rich foods.

Also, drink plenty of water. Dehydration can lead to headaches and exhaustion, especially if your brain is already under stress from the rigors of the test. Particularly if your test is a long one, drink water during the breaks. And if possible, take an energy-boosting snack to eat between sections.

> **Review Video: <u>How Diet Can Affect your Mood</u>**
> Visit mometrix.com/academy and enter code: 624317

Along with sleep and diet, a third important part of physical health is exercise. Maintaining a steady workout schedule is helpful, but even taking 5-minute study breaks to walk can help get your blood pumping faster and clear your head. Exercise also releases endorphins, which contribute to a positive feeling and can help combat test anxiety.

When you nurture your physical health, you are also contributing to your mental health. If your body is healthy, your mind is much more likely to be healthy as well. So take time to rest, nourish your body with healthy food and water, and get moving as much as possible. Taking these physical steps will make you stronger and more able to take the mental steps necessary to overcome test anxiety.

> **Review Video: <u>How to Stay Healthy and Prevent Test Anxiety</u>**
> Visit mometrix.com/academy and enter code: 877894

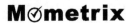

Mental Steps for Beating Test Anxiety

Working on the mental side of test anxiety can be more challenging, but as with the physical side, there are clear steps you can take to overcome it. As mentioned earlier, test anxiety often stems from lack of preparation, so the obvious solution is to prepare for the test. Effective studying may be the most important weapon you have for beating test anxiety, but you can and should employ several other mental tools to combat fear.

First, boost your confidence by reminding yourself of past success—tests or projects that you aced. If you're putting as much effort into preparing for this test as you did for those, there's no reason you should expect to fail here. Work hard to prepare; then trust your preparation.

Second, surround yourself with encouraging people. It can be helpful to find a study group, but be sure that the people you're around will encourage a positive attitude. If you spend time with others who are anxious or cynical, this will only contribute to your own anxiety. Look for others who are motivated to study hard from a desire to succeed, not from a fear of failure.

Third, reward yourself. A test is physically and mentally tiring, even without anxiety, and it can be helpful to have something to look forward to. Plan an activity following the test, regardless of the outcome, such as going to a movie or getting ice cream.

When you are taking the test, if you find yourself beginning to feel anxious, remind yourself that you know the material. Visualize successfully completing the test. Then take a few deep, relaxing breaths and return to it. Work through the questions carefully but with confidence, knowing that you are capable of succeeding.

Developing a healthy mental approach to test taking will also aid in other areas of life. Test anxiety affects more than just the actual test—it can be damaging to your mental health and even contribute to depression. It's important to beat test anxiety before it becomes a problem for more than testing.

> **Review Video: <u>Test Anxiety and Depression</u>**
> Visit mometrix.com/academy and enter code: 904704

Study Strategy

Being prepared for the test is necessary to combat anxiety, but what does being prepared look like? You may study for hours on end and still not feel prepared. What you need is a strategy for test prep. The next few pages outline our recommended steps to help you plan out and conquer the challenge of preparation.

STEP 1: SCOPE OUT THE TEST

Learn everything you can about the format (multiple choice, essay, etc.) and what will be on the test. Gather any study materials, course outlines, or sample exams that may be available. Not only will this help you to prepare, but knowing what to expect can help to alleviate test anxiety.

STEP 2: MAP OUT THE MATERIAL

Look through the textbook or study guide and make note of how many chapters or sections it has. Then divide these over the time you have. For example, if a book has 15 chapters and you have five days to study, you need to cover three chapters each day. Even better, if you have the time, leave an extra day at the end for overall review after you have gone through the material in depth.

If time is limited, you may need to prioritize the material. Look through it and make note of which sections you think you already have a good grasp on, and which need review. While you are studying, skim quickly through the familiar sections and take more time on the challenging parts. Write out your plan so you don't get lost as you go. Having a written plan also helps you feel more in control of the study, so anxiety is less likely to arise from feeling overwhelmed at the amount to cover.

STEP 3: GATHER YOUR TOOLS

Decide what study method works best for you. Do you prefer to highlight in the book as you study and then go back over the highlighted portions? Or do you type out notes of the important information? Or is it helpful to make flashcards that you can carry with you? Assemble the pens, index cards, highlighters, post-it notes, and any other materials you may need so you won't be distracted by getting up to find things while you study.

If you're having a hard time retaining the information or organizing your notes, experiment with different methods. For example, try color-coding by subject with colored pens, highlighters, or post-it notes. If you learn better by hearing, try recording yourself reading your notes so you can listen while in the car, working out, or simply sitting at your desk. Ask a friend to quiz you from your flashcards, or try teaching someone the material to solidify it in your mind.

STEP 4: CREATE YOUR ENVIRONMENT

It's important to avoid distractions while you study. This includes both the obvious distractions like visitors and the subtle distractions like an uncomfortable chair (or a too-comfortable couch that makes you want to fall asleep). Set up the best study environment possible: good lighting and a comfortable work area. If background music helps you focus, you may want to turn it on, but otherwise keep the room quiet. If you are using a computer to take notes, be sure you don't have any other windows open, especially applications like social media, games, or anything else that could distract you. Silence your phone and turn off notifications. Be sure to keep water close by so you stay hydrated while you study (but avoid unhealthy drinks and snacks).

Also, take into account the best time of day to study. Are you freshest first thing in the morning? Try to set aside some time then to work through the material. Is your mind clearer in the afternoon or evening? Schedule your study session then. Another method is to study at the same time of day that you will take the test, so that your brain gets used to working on the material at that time and will be ready to focus at test time.

STEP 5: STUDY!

Once you have done all the study preparation, it's time to settle into the actual studying. Sit down, take a few moments to settle your mind so you can focus, and begin to follow your study plan. Don't give in to distractions or let yourself procrastinate. This is your time to prepare so you'll be ready to fearlessly approach the test. Make the most of the time and stay focused.

Of course, you don't want to burn out. If you study too long you may find that you're not retaining the information very well. Take regular study breaks. For example, taking five minutes out of every hour to walk briskly, breathing deeply and swinging your arms, can help your mind stay fresh.

As you get to the end of each chapter or section, it's a good idea to do a quick review. Remind yourself of what you learned and work on any difficult parts. When you feel that you've mastered the material, move on to the next part. At the end of your study session, briefly skim through your notes again.

But while review is helpful, cramming last minute is NOT. If at all possible, work ahead so that you won't need to fit all your study into the last day. Cramming overloads your brain with more information than it can process and retain, and your tired mind may struggle to recall even previously learned information when it is overwhelmed with last-minute study. Also, the urgent nature of cramming and the stress placed on your brain contribute to anxiety. You'll be more likely to go to the test feeling unprepared and having trouble thinking clearly.

So don't cram, and don't stay up late before the test, even just to review your notes at a leisurely pace. Your brain needs rest more than it needs to go over the information again. In fact, plan to finish your studies by noon or early afternoon the day before the test. Give your brain the rest of the day to relax or focus on other things, and get a good night's sleep. Then you will be fresh for the test and better able to recall what you've studied.

STEP 6: TAKE A PRACTICE TEST

Many courses offer sample tests, either online or in the study materials. This is an excellent resource to check whether you have mastered the material, as well as to prepare for the test format and environment.

Check the test format ahead of time: the number of questions, the type (multiple choice, free response, etc.), and the time limit. Then create a plan for working through them. For example, if you have 30 minutes to take a 60-question test, your limit is 30 seconds per question. Spend less time on the questions you know well so that you can take more time on the difficult ones.

If you have time to take several practice tests, take the first one open book, with no time limit. Work through the questions at your own pace and make sure you fully understand them. Gradually work up to taking a test under test conditions: sit at a desk with all study materials put away and set a timer. Pace yourself to make sure you finish the test with time to spare and go back to check your answers if you have time.

After each test, check your answers. On the questions you missed, be sure you understand why you missed them. Did you misread the question (tests can use tricky wording)? Did you forget the information? Or was it something you hadn't learned? Go back and study any shaky areas that the practice tests reveal.

Taking these tests not only helps with your grade, but also aids in combating test anxiety. If you're already used to the test conditions, you're less likely to worry about it, and working through tests until you're scoring well gives you a confidence boost. Go through the practice tests until you feel comfortable, and then you can go into the test knowing that you're ready for it.

Test Tips

On test day, you should be confident, knowing that you've prepared well and are ready to answer the questions. But aside from preparation, there are several test day strategies you can employ to maximize your performance.

First, as stated before, get a good night's sleep the night before the test (and for several nights before that, if possible). Go into the test with a fresh, alert mind rather than staying up late to study.

Try not to change too much about your normal routine on the day of the test. It's important to eat a nutritious breakfast, but if you normally don't eat breakfast at all, consider eating just a protein bar. If you're a coffee drinker, go ahead and have your normal coffee. Just make sure you time it so that the caffeine doesn't wear off right in the middle of your test. Avoid sugary beverages, and drink enough water to stay hydrated but not so much that you need a restroom break 10 minutes into the test. If your test isn't first thing in the morning, consider going for a walk or doing a light workout before the test to get your blood flowing.

Allow yourself enough time to get ready, and leave for the test with plenty of time to spare so you won't have the anxiety of scrambling to arrive in time. Another reason to be early is to select a good seat. It's helpful to sit away from doors and windows, which can be distracting. Find a good seat, get out your supplies, and settle your mind before the test begins.

When the test begins, start by going over the instructions carefully, even if you already know what to expect. Make sure you avoid any careless mistakes by following the directions.

Then begin working through the questions, pacing yourself as you've practiced. If you're not sure on an answer, don't spend too much time on it, and don't let it shake your confidence. Either skip it and come back later, or eliminate as many wrong answers as possible and guess among the remaining ones. Don't dwell on these questions as you continue—put them out of your mind and focus on what lies ahead.

Be sure to read all of the answer choices, even if you're sure the first one is the right answer. Sometimes you'll find a better one if you keep reading. But don't second-guess yourself if you do immediately know the answer. Your gut instinct is usually right. Don't let test anxiety rob you of the information you know.

If you have time at the end of the test (and if the test format allows), go back and review your answers. Be cautious about changing any, since your first instinct tends to be correct, but make sure you didn't misread any of the questions or accidentally mark the wrong answer choice. Look over any you skipped and make an educated guess.

At the end, leave the test feeling confident. You've done your best, so don't waste time worrying about your performance or wishing you could change anything. Instead, celebrate the successful

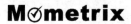

completion of this test. And finally, use this test to learn how to deal with anxiety even better next time.

Important Qualification

Not all anxiety is created equal. If your test anxiety is causing major issues in your life beyond the classroom or testing center, or if you are experiencing troubling physical symptoms related to your anxiety, it may be a sign of a serious physiological or psychological condition. If this sounds like your situation, we strongly encourage you to seek professional help.

Tell Us Your Story

We at Mometrix would like to extend our heartfelt thanks to you for letting us be a part of your journey. It is an honor to serve people from all walks of life, people like you, who are committed to building the best future they can for themselves.

We know that each person's situation is unique. But we also know that, whether you are a young student or a mother of four, you care about working to make your own life and the lives of those around you better.

That's why we want to hear your story.

We want to know why you're taking this test. We want to know about the trials you've gone through to get here. And we want to know about the successes you've experienced after taking and passing your test.

In addition to your story, which can be an inspiration both to us and to others, we value your feedback. We want to know both what you loved about our book and what you think we can improve on.

The team at Mometrix would be absolutely thrilled to hear from you! So please, send us an email at tellusyourstory@mometrix.com or visit us at mometrix.com/tellusyourstory.php and let's stay in touch.

Additional Bonus Material

Due to our efforts to try to keep this book to a manageable length, we've created a link that will give you access to all of your additional bonus material.

Please visit http://www.mometrix.com/bonus948/medicaltech to access the information.